Transfusion in the Year 2020: The Future of Blood Transfusion

Guest Editor

MARK YAZER, MD, FRCPC

CLINICS IN LABORATORY MEDICINE

www.labmed.theclinics.com

Consulting Editor
ALAN WELLS, MD, DMSc

June 2010 • Volume 30 • Number 2

SAUNDERS an imprint of ELSEVIER, Inc.

W.B. SAUNDERS COMPANY
A Division of Elsevier Inc.

1600 John F. Kennedy Boulevard • Suite 1800 • Philadelphia, Pennsylvania 19103-2899

http://www.theclinics.com

CLINICS IN LABORATORY MEDICINE Volume 30, Number 2

June 2010 ISSN 0272-2712, ISBN-13: 978-1-4377-1832-4

Editor: Katie Hartner
Developmental Editor: Donald Mumford

Reprints. For copies of 100 or more, of articles in this publication, please contact the Commercial Reprints Department, Elsevier Inc., 360 Park Avenue South, New York, New York 10010-1710. Tel. (212) 633-3813, Fax: (212) 462-1935, E-mail: reprints@elsevier.com.

Clinics in Laboratory Medicine (ISSN 0272-2712) is published quarterly by Elsevier Inc., 360 Park Avenue South, New York, NY 10010-1710. Months of issue are March, June, September, and December. Business and Editorial offices: 1600 John F. Kennedy Blvd., Suite 1800, Philadelphia, PA 19103-2899. Periodicals postage paid at New York, NY and additional mailing offices. Subscription prices are $220.00 per year (US individuals), $347.00 per year (US institutions), $114.00 (US students), $253.00 per year (Canadian individuals), $438.00 per year (foreign institutions), $157.00 (foreign students). Foreign air speed delivery is included in all *Clinics* subscription prices. All prices are subject to change without notice. POSTMASTER: Send address changes to *Clinics in Laboratory Medicine*, Elsevier Health Sciences Division, Subscription Customer Service, 3251 Riverport Lane, Maryland Heights, MO 63043. **Customer Service: 1-800-654-2452 (US). From outside of the US and Canada, call 1-314-447-8871. Fax: 1-314-447-8029. E-mail: journalscustomerservice-usa@elsevier.com (for print support) or journalsonlinesupport-usa@elsevier.com (for online support).**

Clinics in Laboratory Medicine is covered in *EMBASE/Exerpta Medica*, *MEDLINE/PubMed (Index Medicus)*, *Cinahl, Current Contents/Clinical Medicine, BIOSIS* and *ISI/BIOMED.*

Printed and bound by CPI Group (UK) Ltd, Croydon, CR0 4YY

Transferred to Digital Print 2011

Contributors

GUEST EDITOR

MARK YAZER, MD, FRCPC
Associate Professor of Pathology, University of Pittsburgh Medical Center; Institute for Transfusion Medicine, Pittsburgh, Pennsylvania

AUTHORS

STEWART ABBOT, PHD
Celgene Cellular Therapeutics, Warren, New Jersey

ABDU I. ALAYASH, PhD
Chief, Laboratory of Biochemistry and Vascular Biology, Division of Hematology; Center for Biologics Evaluation and Research, Food and Drug Administration, Rockville Pike, Bethesda, Maryland

DAVID K.C. COOPER, MD, PhD, FRCS
Professor of Surgery, Thomas E. Starzl Transplantation Institute, University of Pittsburgh Medical Center, Pittsburgh, Pennsylvania

GEOFF DANIELS, PhD, FRCPath
Head of Molecular Diagnostics, International Blood Group Reference Laboratory, Bristol Institute for Transfusion Sciences, NHS Blood and Transplant, Filton, Bristol, United Kingdom

DANA V. DEVINE, PhD
Research and Development, Canadian Blood Services; Professor of Pathology and Laboratory Medicine, University of British Columbia Center for Blood Research, Vancouver, British Columbia, Canada

ROGER Y. DODD, PhD
Vice President, American Red Cross, Holland Laboratory, Rockville, Maryland

LUC DOUAY, MD, PhD
Professor of Hematology, Université Pierre et Marie Curie; Head of Laboratory of Hematology, Hôpital Armand Trousseau, Assistance Publique-Hôpitaux de Paris; Scientific Director for Cell Therapy, Etablissement Français du Sang, Paris-Ile de, Paris, France

KIRSTIN FINNING, PhD
Clinical Scientist, International Blood Group Reference Laboratory, Bristol Institute for Transfusion Sciences, NHS Blood and Transplant, Filton, Bristol, United Kingdom

MONIQUE P. GELDERMAN, PhD
Laboratory of Cellular Hematology, Division of Hematology, Office of Blood Research and Review, Center for Biologics Evaluation and Research, Food and Drug Administration, Rockville, Maryland

HANNES HANSEN-MAGNUSSON, MA
Faculty of Social Sciences and Economics, Wissenschaftlicher Mitarbeiter/Lecturer at the Chair for Politics & Global Governance, University of Hamburg, Hamburg, Germany

HIDETAKA HARA, MD, PhD
Research Instructor in Surgery, Thomas E. Starzl Transplantation Institute, University of Pittsburgh Medical Center, Pittsburgh, Pennsylvania

PETE MARTIN
Clinical Scientist, International Blood Group Reference Laboratory, Bristol Institute for Transfusion Sciences, NHS Blood and Transplant, Filton, Bristol, United Kingdom

JOANN M. MOULDS, PhD, MT(ASCP)SBB
Director, Clinical Immunogenetics, LifeShare Blood Centers, Shreveport, Louisiana

KATHERINE SERRANO, PhD
Research and Development, Canadian Blood Services; Research Associate, Pathology and Laboratory Medicine, University of British Columbia Center for Blood Research, Vancouver, British Columbia, Canada

JAROSLAV G. VOSTAL, MD, PhD
Laboratory of Cellular Hematology, Division of Hematology, Office of Blood Research and Review, Center for Biologics Evaluation and Research, Food and Drug Administration, Rockville, Maryland

JONATHAN H. WATERS, MD
Professor and Chief, Department of Anesthesiology, Magee Womens Hospital of University of Pittsburgh Medical Center, Pittsburgh, Pennsylvania

MARK YAZER, MD, FRCPC
Associate Professor of Pathology, University of Pittsburgh Medical Center; Institute for Transfusion Medicine, Pittsburgh, Pennsylvania

JAMES C. ZIMRING, MD, PhD
Associate Professor, Department of Pathology and Laboratory Medicine, Center for Transfusion and Cellular Therapies, Emory University School of Medicine, Atlanta, Georgia

Contents

Preface   xi

Mark Yazer

Genetically Engineered Pigs as a Source for Clinical Red Blood Cell Transfusion   365

David K.C. Cooper, Hidetaka Hara, and Mark Yazer

The transfusion of animal blood or red blood cells (RBCs) into humans goes back to 1667, and the practice persisted until the early 1900s. In recent years, in part because of the shortage of acceptable and safe human blood worldwide, there has been renewed interest in the possibility of using genetically-engineered pigs as sources of RBCs for clinical transfusion. Pigs are becoming available in which the cells, tissues, and organs are to some extent protected from the human immune response. This extends significant protection from antibody-mediated complement lysis. Transfusion of these RBCs into nonhuman primates, however, indicates that they are rapidly lost from the circulation, almost certainly through the phagocytic activity of macrophages. Further genetic manipulation may resolve this problem. In view of the potential advantages of pig RBCs with regard to the absence of infectious microorganisms and the rapid progress being made in genetically modifying pigs, pig RBCs may eventually become a feasible source of blood for clinical transfusion.

Setbacks in Blood Substitutes Research and Development: A Biochemical Perspective   381

Abdu I. Alayash

Recent setbacks in using Hb-based technology to develop oxygen carriers or blood substitutes may spur new and fundamentally different approaches for the development of a new generation of hemoglobin-based oxygen carriers (HBOCs). This article briefly details some underlying mechanisms that may have been responsible for the adverse-event profile associated with HBOCs, with a focus on the contribution of the author's laboratory toward identifying some of these biochemical pathways and some ways and means to control them. It is hoped that this will aid in the development of a safe and effective second generation of HBOCs.

From Stem Cell to Red Blood Cells In Vitro: "The 12 Labors of Hercules"   391

Luc Douay

This article describes the research in progress that will permit the large-scale production of human red blood cells from hematopoietic stem cells. It also discusses the current state of this research, suggests the obstacles to be overcome to pass from the laboratory model to clinical practice, and analyzes the possible indications in the medium and long term. The potential interest of pluripotent stem cells as an unlimited source of red blood cells is considered. If it succeeds, this new approach could mark a considerable advance in the field of transfusion.

The Three "R"s of Blood Transfusion in 2020; Routine, Reliable and Robust   405

Stewart Abbot

To predict the timing and nature of future changes in the practice of blood transfusion, several factors must be considered. The historical rate of change of a scientific field can often provide a rough guide to the rate of future progress. To improve the accuracy of these predictions, historical rates must be adjusted to take into account the decelerating effects of technological or methodological barriers to progress, together with the potentially accelerating effects of transformative technology breakthroughs and unmet needs in the field that act as drivers for change. The cumulative impact of unpredictable and, often, limited availability of traditional blood donors, increasingly elderly populations, the potential for storage-associated adverse events, and increasingly prevalent transfusion-transmittable diseases is likely to provide significant drive to develop transformational alternatives to current transfusion practices. Considering the current stage of development of stem cell–based therapeutics and the rates of change in clinically compatible bioreactors and cell sorting systems, it is reasonable to believe that stem cell–based ex vivo manufacture of blood components will become routine, robust, and reliable within the next decade.

Future of Molecular Testing for Red Blood Cell Antigens   419

Joann M. Moulds

When one looks at the field of molecular pathology or transplantation, it is evident that molecular biology has made a positive impact on medicine. However, the progress in transfusion medicine has been slower and more cautious than in other areas of the clinical laboratory. To understand where the field may go in the next 10 years requires that the reader understand what technology is available now. Therefore, this article discusses the current state of the art for red-cell genotyping and newer, ever-evolving molecular technologies. Because it is impossible to present all of the molecular techniques and their variations in this article, the author selects a group of methodologies to review and speculates where the field of molecular immunohematology may be in 2020.

Noninvasive Fetal Blood Grouping: Present and Future   431

Geoff Daniels, Kirstin Finning, and Pete Martin

Identification of the molecular basis of the D polymorphism of the Rh blood group system in the 1990s made it possible to predict D phenotype from DNA. The most valuable application of this has been the determination of fetal D type in pregnant D-negative women with anti-D. Knowledge of fetal D type reveals whether the fetus is at risk of hemolytic disease of the fetus and newborn so that the pregnancy can be managed appropriately. Noninvasive fetal D typing for D-negative pregnant women with anti-D, performed on the small quantity of fetal DNA present in the blood of pregnant women, is now routine practice in several European countries. Noninvasive fetal blood grouping for C, c, E, and K also may be provided as a routine service for alloimmunized pregnant women. In many countries, all D-negative pregnant women are offered anti-D prophylaxis antenatally, yet in a predominantly Caucasian population, about 38% will be carrying a D-negative fetus and will receive the treatment unnecessarily. Large-scale trials to ascertain the accuracy of high-throughput, automated methods suggest that fetal D screening of all D-negative pregnant women is feasible, and it is likely that fetal D screening in D-negative pregnant women will be policy in some European countries within the next few years.

Current and Future Cellular Transfusion Products   443

Monique P. Gelderman and Jaroslav G. Vostal

Novel red blood cell and platelet transfusion products may be synthetic or may result from modifications to approved collection, processing, and storage procedures for existing cellular products. They must be reviewed and evaluated by the Food and Drug Administration before being legally marketed in the United States to ensure they are safe, pure, and potent. This article reviews the literature and discusses the current and future state of cellular transfusion products.

The Future of Blood Management   453

Jonathan H. Waters

An evolving understanding of the consequences of allogeneic blood transfusion and escalating costs of providing allogeneic blood have resulted in an interest in blood management. Understanding the consequences of allogeneic transfusion includes a recognition of the immunosuppressive effects of allogeneic transfusion, a growing awareness of transfusion-related acute lung injury, and a rediscovery of transfusion-associated circulatory overload. More recently, interest has focused on the effect of stored blood on patient outcome. Although this discussion is not all-inclusive, it is intended to show that many techniques can be applied to decrease the exposure to allogeneic blood.

Recent Developments and Future Directions of Alloimmunization to Transfused Blood Products   467

James C. Zimring

Monitoring and managing alloimmunization are among the primary functions of the clinical transfusion medicine laboratory. However, despite hundreds of different blood group antigens that vary from person to person, only a minority of transfusion recipients become alloimmunized. Currently, there are no tests that predict which patients will become alloimmunized. Moreover, there are no therapeutic interventions to prevent alloimmunization (outside of RhD immune globulin) besides phenotypic matching. Understanding the biologic factors that regulate alloimmunization may allow the generation of clinical tests with predictive capabilities and provide a rational basis for developing therapeutic interventions. This article summarizes recent advances in understanding alloimmunization, with a focus of identifying future directions in laboratory testing and management of transfusion. In addition to analyzing humoral alloimmunization, potential extensions of transfusion medicine to sequelae of cellular immunization are explored.

The Platelet Storage Lesion   475

Dana V. Devine and Katherine Serrano

The gradual loss of quality in stored platelets as measured collectively with various metabolic, functional, and morphologic in vitro assays is known as the platelet storage lesion. With the advent of pathogen reduction technologies and improved testing that can greatly reduce the risk for bacterial contamination, the platelet storage lesion is emerging as the main challenge to increasing the shelf life of platelet concentrates. This article discusses the contribution of platelet production methods to the storage lesion, long-established and newly developed methods used to determine platelet quality, and the significance for clinical transfusion outcome. Highlighted are the novel technologies applied to platelet storage including platelet additive solutions and pathogen inactivation.

Governance in the European Union: The European Blood Directive as an Evolving Practice   489

Hannes Hansen-Magnusson

This article reconstructs governance practices related to blood policy that have developed within in the European Union (EU) over the last 15 years. It describes core aspects of the policy and argues that, despite an integrated cooperative approach between policy-makers and practitioners, this policy remains an open and evolving process. The European Blood Directive (2002/98/EC) and its subsequent directives managed, for the first time, to create an overarching framework for transfusion procedures. This framework consists of a number of standard definitions as well as detailed standard operating procedures, yet leaves room for interpretation and different practices between EU member states. A recently published report on the progress of transposition of the Directives into national legislation reveals different standards, suggesting a lack of uniformity of safety and quality requirements. Further, gaps in the directives amount to practical medical problems, while increased mobility among EU citizens may add further problems to achieving the objective of a self-sufficient supply of blood and blood products. This might undermine public confidence in the quality of blood products and the health protection of donors, which, in turn, must be countered by a cooperative effort of policy-makers and blood establishments.

Emerging Pathogens in Transfusion Medicine   499

Roger Y. Dodd

Although the risk of infection with hepatitis and human immunodeficiency viruses from blood transfusions has been reduced to negligible levels, emerging infections continue to offer threats. Such threats occur with any infection that has an asymptomatic, blood-borne phase. In the past, it was thought that any emerging transfusion-transmitted disease would have epidemiologic properties similar to those of AIDS or viral hepatitis. Over the past 20 years, however, greatest concern has arisen from variant Creutzfeldt-Jakob disease, West Nile virus, and Babesia. These and other emerging infections are discussed in the context of blood safety.

Index   511

FORTHCOMING ISSUES

Prenatal Testing
Anthony Odibo, MD, MSCE,
Guest Editor

Genetics
Alan Wells, MD, DMSc,
Guest Editor

Systems Biology
Zoltan Oltvai, MD,
Guest Editor

Veterinary Testing
Mary Christopher, DVM, PhD,
Dipl ACVP, Dipl ECVCP,
Guest Editor

RECENT ISSUES

March 2010
Emerging Pathogens
A. William Pasculle, ScD,
and James Snyde, PhD,
Guest Editors

December 2009
**Respiratory Viruses in Pediatric
and Adult Populations**
Alexander J. McAdam, MD, PhD,
Guest Editor

September 2009
Point-of-Care Testing
Kent Lewandrowski, MD,
Guest Editor

THE CLINICS ARE NOW AVAILABLE ONLINE!

Access your subscription at:
www.theclinics.com

Preface

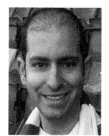

Mark Yazer, MD, FRCPC
Guest Editor

Dear Colleagues,

Welcome to this issue of *Clinics in Laboratory Medicine*, an issue devoted to predicting the future of some different aspects of transfusion medicine. The title, "Transfusion in the Year 2020: The Future of Blood Transfusion," was chosen not just as a play on the optical term for "perfect vision," but because I believe that in the next 10 years significant new advances in technology might change the way transfusion medicine and blood banking are practiced and thought about. Much like other medical specialties, transfusion medicine is a science and an art. The science of blood groups, alloimmunization, transmissible disease testing, and component preparation helps produce blood products that, in many ways, are as safe as they have ever been. The art of transfusion medicine really comes down to knowing when to use these blood products—a platelet count of 15,000/mL might for one patient be perfectly acceptable and not require a transfusion whereas for another patient the same platelet count would justifiably trigger a lifesaving platelet transfusion. Just like the mutual fund ads on TV that remind us to consider the risks and benefits of investing in the stock market, patient-centered transfusion strategies are all about mitigating risk while maximizing the benefits for recipients (and hopefully with greater regularity than Wall Street!). This notion of risk reduction is a recurrent theme in the articles that follow, which can be approximately divided into 2 categories: innovative technologies and innovative paradigms.

One way to avoid certain risks of transfusion, especially that of human-to-human transmissible diseases, is to start with blood products that are less likely to harbor these pathogens in the first place. The first in the set of articles dealing with innovative technologies showcases some of the attempts to derive transfusable blood products from unconventional starting materials. David Cooper, Hidetaka Hara, and I provide a fascinating history of xenotransfusion—transfusing blood from different species of animals—and describe some of our recent in vitro attempts to modify swine red blood cells (RBCs) for human transfusion. Then, Abdu Alayash describes some of the setbacks that have been encountered in trying to produce what are commonly known as blood substitutes and highlights some of the obstacles that need to be overcome in

Clin Lab Med 30 (2010) xi–xiii
doi:10.1016/j.cll.2010.04.002
0272-2712/10/$ – see front matter © 2010 Elsevier Inc. All rights reserved.

labmed.theclinics.com

the production of a clinically suitable oxygen carrier. Next, Luc Douay and Stewart Abbot provide leading-edge insights into the ability to expand stem cells into mature RBCs; think of it, a nearly inexhaustible source of stem cells is discarded with every placenta. These noncontroversial stem cells could be collected from women who have been repeatedly tested and shown to be free of various transmissible diseases; then, using a bioreactor, they would be expanded and matured into functional RBCs suitable for transfusion. The potential for these RBCs is limitless—they could supplement a local hospital's RBC inventory during the traditional lulls in donations around the holidays and in the summer and be lifesaving on the battlefield.

In certain situations, such as patients who receive chronic transfusion therapy or those who have produced an anti-RBC antibody, it is often desirable to provide donor RBC units whose surface phenotype of proteins and carbohydrates are as closely matched as possible to that of the recipient. Although conventional serologic techniques are the current gold standard for antigen typing, there are some significant limitations to their use, such as the lack of availability of Food and Drug Administration (FDA)–approved reagents and the technical difficulty of phenotyping RBCs from recently transfused recipients. To that end, Joann Moulds describes the state of the art in blood group genotyping; this is a particularly relevant topic given the increasing number of testing platforms that are on the market today and the ones that are sure to follow. On the theme of molecular blood group genotyping, Geoff Daniels and colleagues describe a technique that is in widespread use in Europe but has had little penetration in North America. Fetal genotyping from maternal plasma, the ability to derive a fetus' blood group genotype using a sample taken from mother's peripheral vein, for the purpose of quantifying the risk of hemolytic disease of newborns has been shown to be reliable and is not associated with the significant risks that accompany the traditional methods of obtaining fetal DNA. I hope that over the next few years this lifesaving method of deriving fetal DNA becomes more mainstream on the side of the Atlantic where "football" is played with an oblong ball. This section concludes with a thought-provoking article by Monique Gelderman-Fuhrmann and Jaroslav Vostal at the FDA about the regulatory guidelines and certification requirements that these new technologies might encounter as they are brought to market in the United States.

The next section deals with innovative concepts related to the practice of transfusion and is composed of a series of articles that describe current and future ways of dealing with some of the problems faced by transfusion medicine professionals. All of the risks of receiving allogeneic blood (ie, from the blood bank) are avoided if an allogeneic transfusion is not required. Jonathan Waters shares his vision for blood conservation over the next few years and describes ways of reducing the need for allogeneic transfusions by a variety of techniques, including preoperative hemoglobin optimization, intraoperative cell salvage, and the use of point-of-care tests that provide real-time information on hemoglobin and coagulation profiles to guide the ordering of blood products. In vitro, RBCs exist in a milieu with other cells and are always surrounded by a variety of cytokines and other chemical messengers. Up to now it has been unclear why some recipients of cellular blood products become alloimmunized when exposed to foreign RBC antigens whereas most recipients do not produce anti-RBC antibodies. James Zimring and the members of his laboratory are on the vanguard of studying the effects of inflammation on alloimmunization using a unique mouse model and, in his article, he describes the progress that has been made in understanding the modulatory effects of different types of inflammatory mediators on the immune system in mice and humans. Although much has been published about the changes that occur to RBCs during storage (commonly known as the storage lesion), less is known about the changes that platelets undergo during their 5-day shelf life. Dana Devine and her group detail these changes and speculate on what might be done to extend the shelf life of this blood component that is often in short supply. All blood centers are highly cognizant of the balance between recruiting sufficient numbers of donors yet maintaining the safety of the blood supply. As North Americans travel the world, more and more travel deferrals are being imposed due to the emergence of new and potentially transfusion transmissible diseases. Hannes Hansen-Magnusson looks at the European blood donor situation in light of the significant personal mobility afforded to citizens of the European Union (EU); although EU-wide directives for blood donation exist, the instantiation of these policies varies by country as do rates of various transfusion transmissible diseases. In a related article, Roger Dodd analyzes some of the current and emerging pathogens that threaten the blood supply in North America as the number of potentially transfusion transmissible pathogens increases and alternatives to and avoidance of allogeneic transfusion become more and more attractive.

It is always fun to make predictions—let us come back to this issue in 2020 and see how many came true!

Mark Yazer, MD, FRCPC
University of Pittsburgh Medical Center
3636 Boulevard of the Allies
Pittsburgh, PA 15213, USA

E-mail address:
MYazer@itxm.org

Genetically Engineered Pigs as a Source for Clinical Red Blood Cell Transfusion

David K.C. Cooper, MD, PhD, FRCS[a,*], Hidetaka Hara, MD, PhD[a],
Mark Yazer, MD, FRCPC[b,c]

KEYWORDS

- Erythrocytes • Pig • Red blood cells • Xenotransfusion
- Xenotransplantation

The World Health Organization estimates that more that 81 million units of blood are collected globally each year.[1] More than 15 million red blood cell (RBCs) units are collected in the United States, which provides a slim surplus of units on a national level.[2] However, this surplus does not reflect the day-to-day inventory at local blood banks where transient shortages of RBCs can threaten to compromise patient care. Elective surgeries sometimes need to be postponed, particularly during the summer months and holiday periods when the supply of donated blood is reduced. Not only is human blood a scarce resource, it can pose several potential infectious and noninfectious complications to the recipient. Despite donor screening by behavior/exposure questionnaire and increasingly by nucleic acid viral screening processes, the infectious disease transmission risk is not zero.

More recently, because of concerns relating to the increasing incidence of new variant Creutzfeldt-Jakob disease in Europe, eligibility for blood donation has been made more restrictive by the AABB (formerly known as the American Association of Blood Banks) and the US Food and Drug Administration. Individuals who have been resident in the United Kingdom or Europe for certain periods of time may be prevented from donating blood in the United States. In Europe, there is concern that there will be a significant shortage when a test becomes available for prion disease. As additional donor restrictions are implemented and the population ages, the United States and

[a] Department of Surgery, Thomas E. Starzl Transplantation Institute, University of Pittsburgh Medical Center, Starzl Biomedical Science Tower, W1543, 200 Lothrop Street, Pittsburgh, PA 15261, USA
[b] Department of Pathology, University of Pittsburgh Medical Center, Starzl Biomedical Science Tower, S417, 200 Lothrop Street, Pittsburgh, PA 15261, USA
[c] Institute for Transfusion Medicine, 3636 Boulevard of the Allies, Pittsburgh, PA 15213, USA
* Corresponding author.
E-mail address: cooperdk@upmc.edu

Clin Lab Med 30 (2010) 365–380
doi:10.1016/j.cll.2010.02.001
0272-2712/10/$ – see front matter © 2010 Elsevier Inc. All rights reserved.

labmed.theclinics.com

other countries might lose more donors, which could cause greater limitations on the supply of human blood.

In countries where the incidence of human immunodeficiency virus infection is much higher than in the United Sates (eg, sub-Saharan Africa), the shortage of RBCs and the risks of blood transfusion are, of course, significantly greater.

Because of the difficulty and expense of ensuring that human blood is free of any infectious microorganisms, it would be desirable to develop other sources that could replace human blood for transfusion. Although there has been interest in developing blood substitutes, such as perfluorochemicals and hemoglobin derivatives, these have not been entirely successful.

The use of RBCs from animal sources might help increase the supply. Although there may be some benefits from using cows as the source of RBCs, for example, less fragility and possibly weaker human immune responses,[3] for many reasons,[4] pigs have been identified as potential sources of organs and cells for transplantation (xenotransplantation) or transfusion (xenotransfusion) into humans.[5]

XENOTRANSFUSION: HISTORICAL ASPECTS

The transfusion of nonhuman animal blood or RBCs into humans has a long history that has been reviewed comprehensively by Roux and colleagues.[6] The first blood transfusions in humans were xenotransfusions, using a variety of animals as sources. Following initial animal studies in Oxford in 1665 by Richard Lower, who experimented with transfusions between 2 dogs,[7,8] a Frenchman, Jean-Baptiste Denis, physician to King Louis XIV, performed the first documented clinical blood transfusion in 1667.[9] With the help of a surgeon, Paul Emmerez, Denis transfused blood from a lamb into a young man who had been bled repeatedly as treatment of a high fever; the patient reportedly felt better, although he described symptoms and showed signs that would now be recognized as consistent with an acute hemolytic reaction.

Denis and others in Europe performed numerous clinical xenotransfusions in the next few years, although they were temporarily banned in France in 1670. In 1816, however, John Henry Leacock, an Edinburgh physician, demonstrated in animals that the results were best when the transfusion was between animals of the same species[10]; he recommended that patients should receive human blood. The London obstetrician, James Blundell, confirmed this observation in animal experiments and then, in 1829, performed the first recognized allotransfusion in a woman with post-partum hemorrhage at Guy's Hospital.[11] Despite these experimental observations, xenotransfusions continued throughout the nineteenth century until Karl Landsteiner published his landmark paper on the ABO blood groups in 1900.[12]

PIGS AS SOURCES OF RBCs FOR CLINICAL TRANSFUSION

Pig RBCs (pRBCs) share several common characteristics with human RBCs (**Table 1**).[13-17] pRBC diameters and counts are similar, although the average life span of pRBCs is shorter than of human RBCs. The most closely studied pig blood group system is the A-O (H) system, which is loosely related to the human ABO system.[18-20] Pig herds have been developed that are uniformly of blood type O, the human universal RBC donor; thus ABO compatibility between human recipients and pig donors would be assured. Porcine hemoglobin shares 85% sequence identity with its human counterpart, and also demonstrates a similar three-dimensional structure at 2.8 Å resolution.[21] Furthermore, human hemoglobin has been expressed in transgenic pigs, with normal posttranslational modifications and biologic function.[22]

Table 1		
Pig RBCs share many common characteristics with human RBCs		
	Pig	**Human**
RBC volume	56–95 mL/kg	70 mL/kg
RBC count	5.7–6.9 million/μl	4.2–6.2 millon/μl
RBC diameter	4–8 μm	6–8 μm
Lifespan	86 days	120 days
Blood groups	27	30
Hemoglobin	6–18 g/100 mL	12–18 g/100 mL
Hematocrit	38%–50%	35%–45%
Isotonic	0.85% NaCl	0.9% NaCl

Data from Refs.[15–17]

The bank of pRBCs could potentially be inexhaustible, and the absence of human microorganisms could largely be assured. Pig RBCs do not express swine leukocyte antigens,[23] thus reducing immunogenicity, and do not have nuclei that could harbor porcine endogenous retroviruses,[24,25] although these advantages would be reduced by contamination of the product by white blood cells (WBCs).

Ethical aspects of xenotransfusion have been discussed by Roux and colleagues.[26]

IMMUNOLOGIC BARRIERS

Several immunologic problems need to be resolved before pRBCs can be used for clinical transfusion. Pig RBCs express the Galα1,3Gal (Gal) epitope against which humans have natural (preformed) hemolytic antibodies.[27–29] Transfusion of unmodified pRBCs into unmodified primate recipients results in antibody-antigen binding, complement activation, and the immediate lysis of the transfused cells.[28,30] Gal is a terminal oligosaccharide, similar to the A, B, and O saccharides (**Fig. 1**), and is the major target antigen for natural primate antibodies.

Like anti-AB blood type antibodies, anti-Gal antibodies are believed to develop during infancy as a response to colonization of the gastrointestinal tract by various bacterial and viral flora.[31] As in ABO-incompatible organ allotransplants or RBC allotransfusion, expression of Gal results in almost uniform hyperacute rejection when pig cells are transplanted or pRBCs are transfused into humans, apes, or Old World nonhuman primates, as none of these species express Gal and therefore have naturally occurring anti-Gal antibodies.

Gal is produced by the enzyme, α1,3-galactosyltransferase.[27] The relatively recent breeding of pigs homozygous for α1,3-galactosyltransferase gene knockout (GTKO), which therefore do not express Gal, has overcome this barrier.[32,33]

However, additional naturally occurring human anti-nonGal antibodies have been identified, although the cytotoxicity associated with anti-nonGal antibodies is significantly reduced compared with that to anti-Gal antibodies.[34–36] Nevertheless, they can initiate rapid complement-mediated lysis of pig cells in vitro and rejection of pig organs in nonhuman primates. Some of these target antigens on pRBCs, such as N-glycolylneuraminic acid (NeuGc), might pose a barrier to human transfusion.[37]

NeuGc and N-acetylneuraminic acid are the 2 most abundant forms of sialic acid identified in glycoconjugates.[38] NeuGc is present in all mammals (including the great apes and monkeys), with the notable exception of humans.[39,40] The presence of NeuGc epitopes on pig vascular endothelial cells was identified by Bouhours and

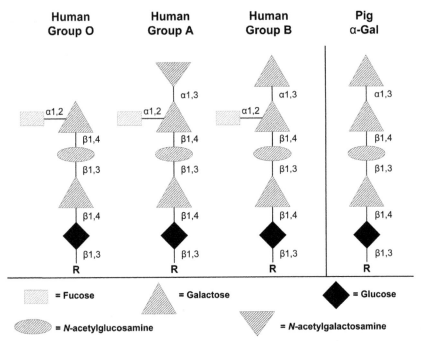

Fig. 1. Carbohydrate structure of human and pig RBCs. Pig RBCs express Gal epitopes on oligosaccharides that are similar in structure to the human blood type B oligosaccharide (which has a fucose side arm). When the terminal Gal epitope is removed from pRBCs, the oligosaccharide is similar to the human blood type O oligosaccharide.

colleagues,[41] in 1996, and its presence on pRBCs was reported by Zhu and Hurst in 2002.[37] These investigators demonstrated that the monosaccharide NeuGc, but not N-acetylneuraminic acid, inhibits approximately 80% of human anti-nonGal antibody binding to pRBCs, suggesting that anti-NeuGc antibody is a major component of anti-nonGal antibodies in most healthy human subjects, at least with regard to pRBCs. Varki's group has provided data to indicate that anti-NeuGc antibodies can be detected in virtually 100% of humans.[40]

If pRBCs are to be transfused successfully into humans, therefore, Gal and NeuGc epitopes probably need to be absent from their cell membranes. In vivo experimental testing of organs and cells from pigs in which the gene for NeuGc has been deleted (NeuGc-KO) may prove difficult as all nonhuman primates and other large experimental animals also express NeuGc, and, therefore, unlike humans, do not make antibodies against this antigen.[40]

Whether there are other terminal oligosaccharides against which humans have natural antibodies remains uncertain. Neither Yeh and colleagues[42] nor Blixt and colleagues[43] were able to identify further saccharides that are definite targets for human anti-pig antibodies, and so the remaining targets for anti-nonGal antibodies could be protein structures. Absence of Gal and NeuGc antigens will almost certainly not completely negate the need for other genetic manipulations of the pig, although further gene knockouts may not be essential. The production of pigs transgenic for a human complement-regulatory protein, such as CD55 (decay-accelerating factor), CD46 (membrane cofactor protein), or CD59 (membrane attack complex-inhibiting protein), may provide sufficient protection from antibody-mediated injury. Even if binding of human antibodies to pig nonGal antigens takes place, the presence of a human complement-regulatory protein may protect the pRBCs from lysis.

INITIAL STUDIES OF pRBC TRANSFUSION IN PRIMATES

Zhu was probably the first to suggest the use of modified pRBCs for clinical transfusion,[15,44,45] and also the first to identify NeuGc as a potential target for human natural anti-nonGal antibodies.[37]

A more detailed investigation of the potential of modified pRBCs for clinical transfusion was performed by Eckermann and colleagues,[17] in 2004. Before GTKO pigs were available, Eckermann and his colleagues followed Zhu's method of treating the pRBCs with the enzyme, α-galactosidase, to remove the Gal epitopes.[46-50] In vitro binding of antibodies in baboon or human sera to untreated/treated pRBCs was assessed by flow cytometry and serum cytotoxicity. In vivo clearance rates of (1) autologous baboon RBCs, (2) unmodified pRBCs, and (3) α-galactosidase-treated pRBCs were measured after transfusion into baboons receiving either no treatment, or depletion of complement[51] $\pm$ depletion of anti-Gal antibodies,[52,53] or of macrophage phagocytes.[54,55]

In vitro binding of baboon or human antibodies to α-galactosidase-treated pRBCs was absent or minimal compared with untreated pRBCs, and serum cytotoxicity was almost completely inhibited. In vivo autologous baboon RBCs survived for more than 16 days and unmodified pRBCs for less than 15 minutes in an untreated baboon.[17] Treated pRBCs survived for 2 hours in an untreated baboon, for 24 hours in a complement-depleted baboon, and for 72 hours when the baboon was depleted of complement and anti-Gal antibody or of complement and macrophage phagocytes. All baboons, however, became sensitized to Gal antigens. Failure to prolong the in vivo survival of treated pRBCs could have been a result of inadequate removal of Gal epitopes, because sensitization to Gal developed, or could have implied other as yet unidentified causes for RBC destruction. α-Galactosidase treatment of pRBCs was therefore clearly inadequate.

However, these initial in vitro studies suggested that α-galactosidase treatment of pRBCs, by removing Gal epitopes, prevented binding of baboon anti-pig antibody and of human anti-Gal antibody to pRBCs. In both cases, this prevented any lysis of the pRBCs, at least in vitro. The inability of α-galactosidase-treated pRBCs to be detected for more than a few hours when infused into a baboon (even when the recipient baboon's complement has been depleted) was initially interpreted as being the effect of macrophage phagocytic activity, possibly following recognition of nonGal porcine antigens. The prolongation of survival of treated pRBCs infused into a baboon in which macrophage phagocytic activity had been suppressed by medronate liposome therapy supported this conclusion. Diminished viability of the pRBCs after α-galactosidase treatment was excluded as a factor in their rapid loss from the circulation by the results of fragility tests that confirmed no difference in fragility between treated and untreated cells.

However, the subsequent sensitization to Gal antigens that developed in all of the baboons exposed to pRBCs indicated that not all Gal had been removed by α-galactosidase treatment. Sensitization to Gal was not accompanied by the development of elicited antibodies to nonGal antigens, presumably in part because of the lack of expression of swine leukocyte antigens on the surface of pRBCs.[23] Although the baboon recipients of pRBCs became sensitized to Gal, no hemolysis of baboon RBCs, no reduction in hematocrit, and no increases in serum bilirubin or lactate dehydrogenase were observed, suggesting a lack of antibody-mediated destruction of baboon RBCs. These observations supported the conclusion that there is no cross-reactivity between anti-pRBC antibody and anti-baboon RBC antibody.

This study also suggested that human serum (which contains natural anti-NeuGc antibodies) was not significantly cytotoxic in vitro either to baboon RBCs (which express NeuGc) or to α-galactosidase-treated pRBCs, which also express NeuGc. However, to ensure an absence of a hemolytic reaction or the development of a high level of anti-NeuGc antibodies, previous treatment of pRBCs with α-galactosidase and neuraminidase would be necessary.

From the same group, Dor and colleagues[56] transfused pRBCs into 2 baboons. Large volumes of RBCs from wild type (ie, unmodified, WT) pigs were transfused into 2 baboons that were depleted of anti-Gal antibodies and complement. (The hematocrits of the baboons were reduced to 12% and 20%, respectively, before the transfusion to facilitate detection of pRBCs). To protect the pRBCs from immediate antibody-dependent complement activation (hyperacute rejection), 48 hours before the pRBC transfusion, cobra venom factor therapy was initiated to deplete complement in the baboon[50] and an infusion of a soluble synthetic Gal conjugate was begun to deplete (or at least bind) anti-Gal antibody.[53] Detection of pRBCs in baboon blood was performed by flow cytometry, the pRBCs being stained with the murine 1AC monoclonal antibody that binds selectively to glycophorin A of pRBCs.[57]

In the first baboon, the pRBC infusions represented approximately 350% of the baboon's initial RBC volume. After 2 transfusions, 70% of the circulating RBCs were pRBCs. For reasons unrelated to the pRBC transfusion, no further follow-up of this baboon was possible.

The second baboon received a total transfusion of 400 mL over 2 days (equivalent to approximately 285% of the baboon's total RBC volume). pRBCs ultimately accounted for more than one-third of the circulating RBCs. However, 12 hours after the last transfusion there were no detectable pRBCs in the blood. The baboon was euthanized and, at necropsy, the spleen was found to be congested and grossly enlarged to approximately 3 times its normal size. Microscopically, extreme congestion was seen and there was evidence of a follicular hyperplasia, strongly suggesting that the pRBCs had been taken up from the circulation by the baboon's spleen. Other organs, including the liver, were normal in size and appearance.

Although these experiments were clearly unsophisticated, some WT pRBCs survived for several hours in the baboon blood that had been depleted of anti-Gal antibody and complement. The experiments indicated that the rapid removal of pRBCs from the blood could be overcome by the transfusion of a large volume of pRBCs, although this was only transient. The conclusion was drawn that the pRBCs had been removed from the blood by macrophages in the spleen (and possibly the liver).

INITIAL STUDIES OF GTKO pRBC TRANSFUSION IN PRIMATES

When GTKO pigs became available, Rouhani and colleagues[58] investigated RBCs from GTKO pigs exposed to sera from naive humans or baboons or from baboons previously sensitized to pig antigens. Immunoglobulin binding was measured by flow cytometry, and cytotoxicity by hemolytic assay. In vivo, relatively small numbers of GTKO pRBCs were transfused into nonsensitized untreated baboons. The survival of pRBCs was detected by flow cytometry.

In vitro, binding of immunoglobulin (Ig)M from naive human or baboon sera was detected on GTKO pRBCs, but was significantly less than binding to WT pRBCs. IgG binding to GTKO pRBCs was absent or minimal. Sera had minimal cytotoxicity to GTKO pRBCs compared with WT pRBCs. As anticipated, sensitized baboon sera demonstrated much higher IgG binding to GTKO pRBCs and increased cytotoxicity, but again this was less than to WT pRBCs. In vivo, the transfusion of relatively small volumes of GTKO pRBCs was followed by detection of the cells in the baboon blood for only 5 minutes. These studies indicated that pRBCs, even from GTKO pigs, are rapidly phagocytosed from the primate circulation by a mechanism not involving anti-Gal antibodies.

The presence of a low level of anti-nonGal antibodies in naive sera explained the IgM binding to GTKO pRBCs seen on flow cytometry. The relative lack of hemolysis associated with this binding, particularly with baboon sera, indicated that these anti-nonGal antibodies were of low cytotoxicity (or, at least, not cytotoxic through the activation of complement). This result correlated with that of McLaren and colleagues[59] who demonstrated that depletion of anti-Gal antibodies from human serum did not abolish all agglutination of pRBCs.

In the case of human sera, the targets for these anti-nonGal antibodies could include NeuGc epitopes, or possibly unknown neoantigens created through the absence of the terminal Gal epitope.[60–62] However, recent studies by Blixt and colleagues[43] and Yeh and colleagues[42] provide no evidence that other likely oligosaccharide epitopes are exposed after GTKO. Furthermore, Long and colleagues[63] have demonstrated in pigs after GTKO that, although there is a greater expression of the O (H) blood group antigen on WBCs and aortic endothelial cells, there is no expression on RBCs. The absence of anti-NeuGc antibodies in baboon serum may account for the reduced cytotoxicity of pRBCs caused by baboon sera compared with that associated with human sera.

In comparison with the unmodified WT pRBCs transfused into untreated baboons by Eckermann and colleagues[17] and Dor and colleagues,[56] in the study by Rouhani and colleagues,[58] no increased survival was documented following the transfusion of GTKO pRBCs. In 1 of these baboons, pRBCs equivalent to almost 20% of the baboon's total RBCs were transfused, and yet none was detectable 5 minutes later. This outcome suggested that the rapid loss of pRBCs is not solely associated with the expression of Gal, but with other features of the pRBCs recognized by the baboon immune system. It appeared likely that rapid phagocytosis by macrophages takes place, particularly by those in the liver (Kupffer cells) and spleen,[64,65] or killing by natural killer cells, or some other as yet unidentified mechanism, occurred.

With the availability of pigs with further genetic manipulations, it has been possible to study this subject in more detail. Long and colleagues[63] performed in vitro studies comparing RBCs from ABO-compatible and ABO-incompatible humans and WT and GTKO pigs that were each tested for hemagglutination, IgM and IgG antibody binding, and complement-dependent cytotoxicity using human serum. Phagocytosis of RBCs by human monocyte-derived macrophages was measured by coculture in the presence of pooled human O serum.

RBCs showed significant differences with regard to hemagglutination, IgM and IgG binding, and complement-dependent cytotoxicity, with ABO-compatible human RBC/plasma pairings clearly demonstrating the most protection, followed by GTKO pRBCs, which were more protected than ABO-incompatible human RBC/plasma combinations or WT pRBCs (**Fig. 2**). In the absence of pooled human O serum, there was no phagocytosis of any RBCs. In the presence of human serum containing anti-A or anti-B antibodies and anti-pig antibodies, phagocytosis of ABO-incompatible human RBCs was greater than of WT pRBCs, which in turn was greater than GTKO pRBCs.

The investigators concluded that GTKO pRBCs were significantly more compatible than ABO-incompatible human RBCs and WT pRBCs, but were not comparable with

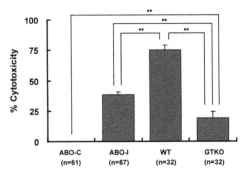

Fig. 2. Human serum complement-dependent cytoxicity (CDC) of ABO-compatible human RBCs (ABO-C), ABO-incompatible human RBCs (ABO-I), wild type pRBCs (WT), and GTKO pRBCs (GTKO). Human sera (50%) of blood types O (n = 10), A (n = 9), B (n = 8), and AB (n = 4) were tested for CDC of ABO-C, ABO-I, WT, and GTKO RBCs. There was significantly greater lysis of WT than of ABO-I and GTKO RBCs ($P<.01$). ABO-I RBCs sustained significantly greater lysis than GTKO RBCs ($P<.01$), but there was significantly greater lysis of GTKO than of ABO-C RBCs ($P<.01$). (**$P<.01$). (*Reproduced from* Long C, Hara H, Pawlikowski Z, et al. Genetically-engineered pig red blood cells for clinical transfusion: initial in vitro studies. Transfusion 2009;49:2423; with permission.)

ABO-compatible human combinations. In the presence of antibody, human mono-cyte-derived macrophages phagocytosed ABO-incompatible human RBC/sera combinations more efficiently than pRBCs.

Monocyte-derived macrophages may have less phagocytic activity than tissue macrophages, (eg, liver or splenic macrophages). However, in the presence of human group O serum, the macrophages phagocytosed the human RBCs more efficiently than WT and GTKO pRBCs (**Fig. 3**). This result was surprising because IgG binding to pRBCs, especially to WT pRBCs, was significantly greater than to the human RBCs used in these experiments.

In the presence of serum from baboons sensitized to GTKO pig organs, however, there was much greater phagocytosis of pRBCs, but less of the human RBCs (see **Fig. 3**). In this case, GTKO and WT pRBCs were phagocytosed equally. Differences between anti-A or anti-B and anti-pig antibodies, therefore, seem to be important in stimulating phagocytosis. Differences in affinity and/or specificity of anti-A or anti-B binding to cells of the same species, and of anti-Gal binding to cells of a different species may also be factors in determining the extent of phagocytosis.

POTENTIAL FUTURE INVESTIGATIONS

Potential mechanisms to overcome the barriers to the xenotransfusion of pRBCs into humans might include creating GTKO pigs that are transgenic for human proteins, such as CD47[66–69] because interspecies CD47 incompatibility may contribute to the phagocytosis of xenogeneic cells by human macrophages.[69] Transfection of cells with the genes for CD47 from the same species as the recipient macrophages prevents phagocytosis by activation of signal regulatory protein α (SIRP α) in mice[70] and humans.[71]

In the study by Long and colleagues,[63] however, in the presence of human group O serum, phagocytosis of human ABO-incompatible RBCs was greater than of the pRBCs, even though IgG binding was greater to the pRBCs. This suggested that anti-body specificity may be a more important factor than the species-related CD47-signal

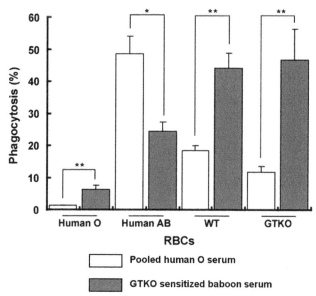

Fig. 3. Phagocytosis of pig RBCs was significantly increased by GTKO-sensitized baboon serum. Human monocyte-derived macrophages and CFSE-labeled RBCs from humans of blood types O and AB and from WT and GTKO pigs were cocultured for 3 hours with heat-inactivated pooled human O serum (*white bars*) or heat-inactivated GTKO-sensitized baboon serum (ie, serum from a baboon that had been sensitized to nonGal antigens following the transplantation of a GTKO pig organ) (*gray bars*). When pooled human O serum was used in the assay, ABO-incompatible human RBCs underwent greater phagocytosis than pRBCs (*white bars*). GTKO-sensitized baboon serum increased phagocytosis of pRBCs, but reduced phagocytosis of human AB RBCs (*gray bars*). The small increase in phagocytosis of human O RBCs is probably related to binding of baboon anti-human antibodies to the RBCs. (*P<.05, **P<.01). (*Reproduced from* Long C, Hara H, Pawlikowski Z, et al. Genetically-engineered pig red blood cells for clinical transfusion: initial in vitro studies. Transfusion 2009;49:2426; with permission.)

regulatory protein α interaction in determining the extent of antibody-dependent phagocytosis. Although a difficult end to achieve, depletion of natural IgG antibodies and prevention of sensitization may be important in preventing antibody-dependent phagocytosis.

GTKO pigs expressing H-transferase were available to this group, but it was determined that the promoter that had been used did not result in expression on the RBCs although there was high expression on WBCs and other tissues (**Fig. 4**). Similarly, WT or GTKO pigs expressing high levels of the complement-regulatory protein, CD46, on WBCs and aortic endothelial cells did not express this transgene on pRBCs. The lack of expression of the H antigen and of CD46 on the RBCs is almost certainly related to the H2K promoter used in the genetic manipulation of the pigs. H2K is a major histocompatibility complex (MHC) Class I promoter, but MHC Class I is not expressed in RBCs. Modifications in the methodology of transgenesis will have to be made if pRBCs are to be protected from antibody-dependent complement-mediated cytotoxicity.

With regard to sensitization to pRBCs, in particular whether this might result in the generation of antibodies that might cross-react with allo-antigens (and thus, for

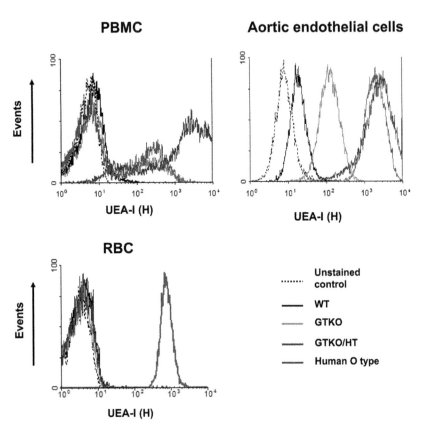

Fig. 4. RBCs from GTKO pigs transgenic for H-transferase (GTKO/HT) did not express the H antigen. Expression of H (blood type O) on peripheral blood mononuclear cells (PBMC), aortic endothelial cells, and RBCs from WT, GTKO, and GTKO/HT pigs and humans (of blood type O) were tested by staining with UEA-1. Dotted lines, unstained or isotype control; black lines, WT cells; red lines, GTKO cells; blue lines, GTKO/HT cells; purple lines, human cells. GTKO/HT PBMC and aortic endothelial cells expressed high levels of H antigen on their surfaces compared with humans and GTKO and WT pigs. GTKO aortic endothelial cells also expressed a significant level. However, although human blood type O RBCs expressed high levels of H antigen, WT, GTKO, and GTKO/HT pRBCs did not express the H antigen.

example, be detrimental to or prevent subsequent human blood transfusions), the current evidence, although limited, is that this would not happen (reviewed in Ref.[72]). Furthermore, the genetic expression of an immunosuppressive transgene, such as CTLA4-Ig[73] on the pRBCs may not only prevent rejection but also protect against the development of T cell–mediated elicited antibodies.

In summary, therefore, in addition to expression of human CD47 (to inhibit antibody-independent and possibly antibody-dependent phagocytosis by macrophages),[70,71] the genetic modifications that may be required for successful pig-to-human RBC xenotransfusion include the expression of (1) the H antigen (to reduce human anti-nonGal binding),[74–79] (2) a human complement-regulatory protein, such as CD46 or CD55 (to protect against complement-dependent cytotoxicity),[80–84] and (3) a gene for the costimulation-blockade molecule, CTLA4-Ig (to suppress T-cell activation and thus prevent sensitization and the production of anti-pig elicited antibody).[73,85–87]

Furthermore knockout of the gene that leads to the expression of NeuGc might confer additional protection against naturally occurring human anti-nonGal antibodies.[37,88]

Other obstacles that will have to be overcome before pig xenotransfusion becomes a reality include (1) demonstrating the complete absence of the transfer of a zoonosis from pRBCs, (2) demonstrating that the breakdown products of pRBCs do not generate immunologically reactive molecules in the recipient that could prevent repeat pRBC transfusions or subsequent human RBC transfusions, (3) determining whether such factors as small differences in isotonicity may affect pRBC survival, and (4) determining the duration and optimal conditions for pRBC storage. Furthermore, society as a whole will have to weigh the potential benefits of pRBC transfusion against any cultural mores that might exist against this treatment modality.

ALTERNATIVE STRATEGIES

A form of chemical camouflage, in which methoxy-polyethylene glycol (mPEG) is covalently bound to the surface of RBCs (from whatever source) through cyanuric chloride coupling has been explored by Jeong and Scott and their respective colleagues.[89–95] This was associated with a profound decrease in anti-blood group antibody binding, and reduced phagocytosis of the coated RBCs from xenogeneic sources. mPEG-treated RBCs are reported to be morphologically normal, have normal osmotic fragility, and normal survival, even after repeated transfusions.[90] After intraperitoneal transfusion into mice, mPEG-treated sheep RBCs showed up to 360-fold improved survival compared with untreated sheep RBCs. This group also reported normal hemoglobin oxidation state, oxygen binding, and cellular deformity, with no sensitization after repeated transfusions.[93] The investigators suggested that the mechanisms underlying mPEG-mediated immunocamouflage are loss of antigen recognition, impaired cell-cell interaction and an ability of endogenous antibodies to effectively recognize and bind foreign antigens.[94]

Having demonstrated that there is considerable variation in expression of Gal on pRBCs (and platelets),[59] McAlister's group demonstrated that mPEG-coating of pRBCs was not as effective as α-galactosidase treatment in reducing hemagglutination of pRBCs by human sera.[30] When the 2 techniques were combined, however, they were more effective than either alone.[30]

The use of PEG to create stealth human RBCs has been met with limited success due in part to anti-PEG antibodies (reviewed in Ref.[95]). Thus, the mPEG technique may have potential in xenotransfusion if these immunologic barriers can be overcome, although multiple genetic modifications in pigs may abrogate the need for such camouflage.

In summary, therefore, we suggest that the genetic modification of pigs has considerable potential in providing an almost unlimited supply of functional RBCs that are protected from the human immune response. With increasing concern about the infectious complications of human-source blood products, pRBCs may eventually resolve the worldwide shortage of human RBCs for clinical transfusion.

ACKNOWLEDGMENTS

The authors thank the many colleagues who have collaborated in these studies over several years, and particularly our colleagues at Revivicor, Inc, Blacksburg, Virginia, who have pioneered the field of the genetic engineering of pigs.

REFERENCES

1. Olsson ML, Clausen H. Modifying the red cell surface: towards an ABO-universal blood supply. Br J Haematol 2008;140:3–12.
2. Whitaker B, Sullivan M. The 2007 nationwide blood collection and utilization survey report. Washington, DC: Department of Health and Human Services; 2008.
3. Johnstone JE, Maclaren LA, Doucet J, et al. In vitro studies regarding the feasibility of bovine erythrocyte xenotransfusion. Xenotransplantation 2004;11:11–7.
4. Cooper DKC, Gollackner B, Sachs DH. Will the pig solve the transplantation backlog? Annu Rev Med 2002;53:133–47.
5. Cooper DKC, Lanza RP. Xeno – the promise of transplanting animal organs into humans. New York: Oxford University Press; 2000. p. 1–274.
6. Roux FA, Sai P, Deschamps JY. Xenotransfusions, past and present. Xenotransplantation 2007;14:208–16.
7. Lower R. The method observed in transfusing the blood out of one live animal into another. Monday December 17, 1666. Philos Trans R Soc Lond A 1666;1:353–8.
8. Lower R. Tractatus de corde. London: Danielem Elzevirium; 1669.
9. Denis JB. Copie d'une lettre e crite a Monsieur de Montmor touchant une nouvelle maniere de gue rir plusieurs maladies par la transfusion du sang, confirme e par deux experiences faites sur des hommes. Le 15 juin 1667. Paris: Jean Cusson; 1667.
10. Schmidt PJ, Leacock AG. Forgotten transfusion history: John Leacock of Barbados. BMJ 2002;325:1485–7.
11. Blundell J. Successful case of transfusion. Lancet 1829;1:431–2.
12. Landsteiner K. Zur Kentniss der antifermentativen lytischen und agglutinierenden Wirkungen des Blutserums und der Lymphe. Zentralblatt für Bakteriologie 1900;28:357–62 [in German].
13. Pond WG, Houpt KA. The biology of the pig. Ithaca (NY): Comstock Pub Associates; 1978.
14. Jandl JH. Blood: textbook of hematology. Boston: Little, Brown; 1996.
15. Zhu A. Introduction to porcine red blood cells: implications for xenotransfusion. Semin Hematol 2000;37:143–9.
16. Cooper DKC. Porcine red blood cells as a source of blood transfusion in humans. Xenotransplantation 2003;10:384–6.
17. Eckermann JM, Buhler LH, Zhu A, et al. Initial investigation of the potential of modified porcine erythrocytes for transfusion in primates. Xenotransplantation 2004;11:18–26.
18. Sako F, Gasa S, Makita A, et al. Human blood group glycosphingolipids of porcine erythrocytes. Arch Biochem Biophys 1990;278:228–37.
19. Smith DM, Newhouse M, Naziruddin B, et al. Blood groups and transfusions in pigs. Xenotransplantation 2006;13:186–94.
20. Yamamoto F, Yamamoto M. Molecular genetic basis of porcine histo-blood group AO system. Blood 2001;97:3308–10.
21. Katz DS, White SP, Huang W, et al. Structure determination of aquomet porcine hemoglobin at 2.8A resolution. J Mol Biol 1994;244:541–53.
22. Rao MJ, Schneider K, Chait BT, et al. Recombinant hemoglobin A produced in transgenic swine: structural equivalence with human hemoglobin A. Artif Cells Blood Substit Immobil Biotechnol 1994;22:695–700.
23. Oostingh GJ, Davies HFS, Tang KCG, et al. Sensitization to swine leukocyte antigens in patients with broadly reactive HLA specific antibodies. Am J Transplant 2002;2:267–73.

24. Patience C, Takeuchi Y, Weiss RA. Zoonosis in xenotransplantation. Curr Opin Immunol 1998;10:539–42.
25. Blusch JH, Patience C, Martin U. Pig endogenous retroviruses and xenotransplantation. Xenotransplantation 2002;9:242–51.
26. Roux FA, Sai P, Deschamps J-Y. Some ethical issues regarding xenotransfusion. Xenotransplantation 2007;14:217–21.
27. Galili U, Shohet SB, Kobrin E, et al. Man, apes, and Old World monkeys differ from other mammals in the expression of alpha-galactosyl epitopes on nucleated cells. J Biol Chem 1988;263:17755–62.
28. Cooper DKC. Depletion of natural antibodies in nonhuman primates – a step towards successful discordant xenografting in man. Clin Transplant 1992;6:178–83.
29. Good AH, Cooper DK, Malcolm AJ, et al. Identification of carbohydrate structures that bind human antiporcine antibodies: implications for discordant xenografting in humans. Transplant Proc 1992;24:559–62.
30. Doucet J, Gao ZH, MacLaren LA, et al. Modification of xenoantigens on porcine erythrocytes for xenotransfusion. Surgery 2004;135:178–86.
31. Galili U, Mandrell RE, Hamadeh RM, et al. Interaction between human natural anti-α-galactosyl immunogloulin G and bacteria of the human flora. Infect Immun 1988;56:1730–7.
32. Phelps CJ, Koike C, Vaught TD, et al. Production of alpha 1,3-galactosyltransferase-deficientpigs. Science 2003;299:411–4.
33. Kolber-Simonds D, Lai L, Watt SR, et al. Production of alpha-1,3-galactosyltransferase null pigs by means of nuclear transfer with fibroblasts bearing loss of heterozygosity mutations. Proc Natl Acad Sci U S A 2004;101:7335–40.
34. Hara H, Ezzelarab M, Rood PP, et al. Allosensitized humans are at no greater risk of humoral rejection of GT-KO pig organs than other humans. Xenotransplantation 2006;13:357–65.
35. Rood PPM, Hara H, Busch JL, et al. Incidence and cytotoxicity of antibodies in cynomolgus monkeys directed to nonGal antigens, and their relevance for experimental models. Transpl Int 2006;19:158–65.
36. Ezzelarab M, Hara H, Busch J, et al. Antibodies directed to pig non-Gal antigens in naive and sensitized baboons. Xenotransplantation 2006;13:400–7.
37. Zhu A, Hurst R. Anti-N-glycolylneuraminic acid antibodies identified in healthy human serum. Xenotransplantation 2002;9:376–81.
38. Schauer R. Sialic acids, chemistry, metabolism, and function. Vienna (Austria): Springer; 1982.
39. Asaoka H, Matsuda H. Detection of N-glycolylneuraminic acid-containing glycoproteins from various animal erythrocytes by chicken monoclonal antibody against Hanganutziu-Deicher antigens. J Vet Med Sci 1994;56:375–7.
40. Varki A. Loss of N-glycolylneuraminic acid in humans: mechanisms, consequences, and implications for hominid evolution. Am J Phys Anthropol 2001;116(Suppl 33):54–69.
41. Bouhours D, Pourcel C, Bouhours JE. Simultaneous expression by porcine aorta endothelial cells of glycosphingolipids bearing the major epitope for human xenoreactive antibodies (Gal alpha 1–3Gal), blood group H determinant and N-glycolylneuraminic acid. Glycoconj J 1996;13:947–53.
42. Yeh P, Ezzelarab M, Bovin N, et al. Investigation of potential carbohydrate antigen targets for human and baboon antibodies. Xenotransplantation, in press.
43. Blixt O, Kumagai-Braesch M, Tibell A, et al. Anticarbohydrate antibody repertoires in patients transplanted with fetal pig islets revealed by glycan arrays. Am J Transplant 2009;9:83–90.

44. Zhu A. Binding of human natural antibodies to nonαGal xenoantigens on porcine erythrocytes. Transplantation 2000;69:2422–8.

45. Zhu A, Hurst R. Human natural antibodies that recognize nonalphaGal antigens on porcine red blood cells. Transplant Proc 2000;32:872–3.

46. Zhu A, Goldstein J. Cloning and functional expression of a cDNA encoding coffee bean alpha-galactosidase. Gene 1994;140:227–31.

47. Zhu A, Monahan C, Zhang Z, et al. High-level expression and purification of coffee bean alpha-galactosidase produced in the yeast *Pichia pastoris*. Arch Biochem Biophys 1995;324:65–70.

48. Zhu A, Wang ZK. Expression and characterization of recombinant alpha-galacto-sidase in baculovirus-infected insect cells. Eur J Biochem 1996;235:332–7.

49. LaVecchio JA, Dunne AD, Edge AS. Enzymatic removal of alpha-galactosyl epitopes from porcine endothelial cells diminishes the cytotoxic effect of natural antibodies. Transplantation 1995;60:841–7.

50. Luo Y, Wen J, Luo C, et al. Pig xenogeneic antigen modification with green coffee bean α-galactosidase: working conditions and potential application in xenotrans-plantation. Xenotransplantation 1999;6:238–48.

51. Kobayashi T, Taniguchi S, Neethling FA, et al. Delayed xenograft rejection of pig-to-baboon cardiac transplants after cobra venom factor therapy. Transplanta-tion 1997;64:1255.

52. Xu Y, Lorf T, Sablinski T, et al. Removal of anti-porcine natural antibodies from human and nonhuman primate plasma in vitro and in vivo by a Galα1-3Galα 1-4αGlc-X immunoaffinity column. Transplantation 1998;65:172–9.

53. Kuwaki K, Knosalla C, Dor FJ, et al. Suppression of natural and elicited antibodies in pig-to-baboon heart transplantation using a human anti-human CD154 mAb based regimen. Am J Transplant 2004;4:363–72.

54. Basker M, Alwayn IP, Buhler L, et al. Clearance of mobilized porcine peripheral blood progenitor cells is delayed by depletion of the phagocytic reticuloendothe-lial system in baboons. Transplantation 2001;72:1278–85.

55. Tseng Y-L, Sachs DH, Cooper DKC. Porcine hematopoietic progenitor cell transplan-tation in nonhuman primates: a review of progress. Transplantation 2005;79:1–9.

56. Dor FJ, Rouhani FJ, Cooper DK. Transfusion of pig red cells into baboons. Xen-otransplantation 2004;11:295–7.

57. Llanes D, Nogal ML, Prados F, et al. An erythroid species-specific antigen of swine detected by a monoclonal antibody. Hybridoma 1992;11:757–64.

58. Rouhani FJ, Dor FJ, Cooper DK. Investigation of red blood cells from alpha1,3-galactosyltransferase-knockout pigs for human blood transfusion. Transfusion 2004;44:1004–12.

59. MacLaren LA, Riggs CM, Johnstone JE, et al. Evaluating porcine RBC and platelet alpha-galactosyl expression. Transfusion 2002;42:1184–8.

60. Cooper DKC. Xenoantigens and xenoantibodies. Xenotransplantation 1998;5: 6–17.

61. Ezzelarab M, Ayares D, Cooper DK. Carbohydrates in xenotransplantation. Immunol Cell Biol 2005;83:396–404.

62. Huflejt ME, Vuskovic M, Vasiliu D, et al. Anti-carbohydrate antibodies of normal sera: findings, surprises and challenges. Mol Immunol 2009;46:3037–49.

63. Long C, Hara H, Pawlikowski Z, et al. Genetically-engineered pig red blood cells for clinical transfusion: initial in vitro studies. Transfusion 2009;49:2418–29.

64. Rees MA, Butler AJ, Negus MC, et al. Classical pathway complement destruction is not responsible for the loss of human erythrocytes during porcine liver perfusion. Transplantation 2004;77:1416–23.

65. Rees MA, Butler AJ, Brons IG, et al. Evidence of macrophage receptors capable of direct recognition of xenogeneic epitopes without opsonization. Xenotransplantation 2005;12:13–9.
66. Oldenborg PA, Zheleznyak A, Fang YF, et al. Role of CD47 as a marker of self on red blood cells. Science 2000;288:2051–4.
67. Oldenborg PA, Gresham HD, Lindberg FP. CD47-signal regulatory protein alpha (SIRPalpha) regulates Fcgamma and complement receptor-mediated phagocytosis. J Exp Med 2001;193:855–62.
68. Vernon-Wilson EF, Kee WJ, Willis AC, et al. CD47 is a ligand for rat macrophage membrane signal regulatory protein SIRP (OX41) and human SIRPalpha 1. Eur J Immunol 2000;30:2130–7.
69. Ide K, Ohdan H, Kobayashi T, et al. Antibody- and complement-independent phagocytotic and cytolytic activities of human macrophages toward porcine cells. Xenotransplantation 2005;12:81–8.
70. Wang H, VerHalen J, Madariaga ML, et al. Attenuation of phagocytosis of xenogeneic cells by manipulating CD47. Blood 2007;109:836–42.
71. Ide K, Wang H, Tahara H, et al. Role for CD47-SIRPalpha signaling in xenograft rejection by macrophages. Proc Natl Acad Sci U S A 2007;104:5062–6.
72. Cooper DKC, Tseng YL, Saidman SL. Alloantibody and xenoantibody cross-reactivity in transplantation. Transplantation 2004;77:1–5.
73. Phelps C, Ball S, Vaught T, et al. Production and characterization of transgenic pigs expressing porcine CTLA4-Ig. Xenotransplantation 2009;16:477–85.
74. Koike C, Kannagi R, Takuma Y, et al. Introduction of [alpha](1,2)- fucosyltransferase and its effect on [alpha]-Gal epitopes in transgenic pig. Xenotransplantation 1996;3:81–6.
75. Sharma A, Okabe J, Birch P, et al. Reduction in the level of Gal(alpha1,3)Galα1,3-Gal (Gal) in transgenic mice and pigs by the expression of an alpha(1,2)fucosyltransferase. Proc Natl Acad Sci U S A 1996;93:7190–5.
76. Osman N, Mckenzie IF, Ostenried K, et al. Combined transgenic expression of alpha-galactosidase and alpha1,2-fucosyltransferase leads to optimal reduction in the major xenoepitope Gal alpha(1,3)Gal. Proc Natl Acad Sci U S A 1997;94:14677–82.
77. Chen CG, Salvaris EJ, Romanella M, et al. Transgenic expression of human alpha1,2-fucosyltransferase (H-transferase) prolongs mouse heart survival in an ex vivo model of xenograft rejection. Transplantation 1998;65:832–7.
78. Costa C, Zhao L, Burton WV, et al. Expression of the human alpha1,2-fucosyltransferase in transgenic pigs modifies the cell surface carbohydrate phenotype and confers resistance to human serum-mediated cytolysis. FASEB J 1999;13:1762–73.
79. Ramsoondar JJ, Machaty Z, Costa C, et al. Production of alpha 1,3- galactosyltransferase-knockout cloned pigs expressing human alpha 1,2-fucosylosyltransferase. Biol Reprod 2003;69:437–45.
80. Cozzi E, White DJG. The generation of transgenic pigs as potential organ donors for humans. Nat Med 1995;1:964–9.
81. Diamond LE, Quinn CM, Martin MJ, et al. A human CD46 transgenic pig model system for the study of discordant xenotransplantation. Transplantation 2001;71:132–42.
82. Adams DH, Kadner A, Chen RH, et al. Human membrane cofactor protein (MCP, CD 46) protects transgenic pig hearts from hyperacute rejection in primates. Xenotransplantation 2001;8:36–40.

83. Loveland BE, Milland J, Kyriakou P, et al. Characterization of a CD46 transgenic pig and protection of transgenic kidneys against hyperacute rejection in non-immunosuppressed baboons. Xenotransplantation 2004;11:171–83.

84. Hara H, Long C, Lin YJ, et al. In vitro investigation of pig cells for resistance to human antibody-mediated rejection. Transpl Int 2008;21:1163–74.

85. Tadaki DK, Craighead N, Saini A, et al. Costimulatory molecules are active in the human xenoreactive T-cell response but not in natural killer-mediated cytotoxicity. Transplantation 2000;70:162–7.

86. Vaughan AN, Malde P, Rogers NJ, et al. Porcine CTLA4-Ig lacks a MYPPPY motif, binds inefficiently to human B7 and specifically suppresses human CD4+ T cell responses costimulated by pig but not human B7. J Immunol 2000;165:3175–81.

87. Mirenda V, Golshayan D, Read J, et al. Achieving permanent survival of islet xenografts by independent manipulation of direct and indirect T-cell responses. Diabetes 2005;54:1048–55.

88. Miwa Y, Kobayashi T, Nagasaka T, et al. Are N-glycolylneuraminic acid (Hanga-nutziu-Deicher) antigens important in pig-to-human xenotransplantation? Xenotransplantation 2004;11:247–53.

89. Jeong ST, Byun SM. Decreased agglutinability of methoxy-polyethylene glycol attached red blood cells: significance as a blood substitute. Artif Cells Blood Substit Immobil Biotechnol 1996;24:503–11.

90. Scott MD, Murad KL, Koumpouras F, et al. Chemical camouflage of antigenic determinants: stealth erythrocytes. Proc Natl Acad Sci U S A 1997;94:7566–71.

91. Scott MD, Bradley AJ, Murad KL. Camouflaged blood cells: low-technology bioengineering for transfusion medicine? Transfus Med Rev 2000;14:53–63.

92. Scott MD, Chen AM. Beyond the red cell: pegylation of other blood cells and tissues. Transfus Clin Biol 2004;11:40–6.

93. Murad KL, Mahany KL, Brugnara C, et al. Structural and functional consequences of antigenic modulation of red blood cells with methoxypoly (ethylene glycol). Blood 1999;93:2121–7.

94. Chen AM, Scott MD. Current and future applications of immunological attenuation via pegylation of cells and tissues. BioDrugs 2001;15:833–47.

95. Garrity G. Modulating the red cell membrane to produce universal/stealth donor red cells suitable for transfusion. Vox Sang 2008;94:87–95.

Setbacks in Blood Substitutes Research and Development: A Biochemical Perspective

Abdu I. Alayash, PhD[a,b,*]

KEYWORDS

• Blood substitutes • Hemoglobin toxicity • Oxygen transport

Blood transfusion in the United States is considered a safe practice although there have been some concerns in recent years, particularly with the emergence of the AIDs epidemic and concerns that donated blood could be contaminated with HIV and other infectious agents. Additionally, the military interest in readily available product encouraged the development of alternatives to donated blood even further. The idea of using blood substitutes in transfusion was first advanced in the 17th century and has continued to fascinate researchers.[1] Growing interest in blood substitutes has resulted in several products that could potentially revolutionize the practice of blood transfusion. Shelf-stable, portable, one-type-fits-all blood substitutes have long held theoretical promise as replacements for standard blood transfusions in extreme, life-threatening situations, such as trauma.

Oxygen therapeutics using hemoglobin-based technology, also known as hemoglobin (Hb)-based oxygen carriers (HBOCs) or blood substitutes, have been under active development for almost 30 years, yet no clinically viable product has been approved. Recently, interest in developing these products has stalled because of problems with product safety (eg, hypertension and oxidative injury) and efficacy (eg, inappropriate oxygen carrying kinetics).[2] Complex biochemical changes introduced onto the Hb molecule caused by chemical or genetic modifications presented a barrier to the full understanding of how these complex molecules operate in a

The findings and conclusions in this article have not been formally disseminated by the Food and Drug Administration and should not be construed to represent any agency determination or policy.

[a] Division of Hematology, Laboratory of Biochemistry and Vascular Biology, USA
[b] Center for Biologics Evaluation and Research, Food and Drug Administration, CBER, FDA, NIH Building 29, Room 112, 8800 Rockville Pike, Bethesda, MD 20892, USA
* Division of Hematology, Laboratory of Biochemistry and Vascular Biology.
E-mail address: abdu.alayash@fda.hhs.gov

Clin Lab Med 30 (2010) 381–389
doi:10.1016/j.cll.2010.02.009
0272-2712/10/$ – see front matter. Published by Elsevier Inc.

cell-free environment. Hemodynamic imbalances as manifested in blood pressure elevation in response to HBOC infusion are viewed by many as a critical step in nitric oxide (NO) modulation, which triggers downstream effects. Other, less-studied enzymatic activities initiated by endogenous oxidants as they react with the heme moiety of Hb may have more lasting tissue-damaging effects than the removal of NO, an autacoid that acts mainly in the microenvironment of cells.[3] Altogether the multiplicity and the disparate of these biochemical hypotheses and conflicting experimental data may have complicated the interpretation of preclinical animal models that have failed to predict the adverse outcome, as frequently observed in the clinical investigations of these therapeutics.[2]

This article briefly details some underlying mechanisms that may have been responsible for the adverse-event profile associated with HBOCs, with a focus on the contribution of the author's laboratory toward identifying some of these biochemical pathways and some ways and means to control them. It is hoped that this will aid in the development of a safe and effective second generation of HBOCs.

BIOCHEMICAL ENGINEERING AND CHARACTERIZATION OF HEMOGLOBIN-BASED OXYGEN CARRIERS

Hemoglobin-based oxygen carriers are prepared predominantly via chemical modification of hemoglobin isolated from outdated human or bovine blood. The manufacturing methods currently employed by industry invariably generate heterogeneous mixtures of polymeric/conjugated species with variable sites of chemical modification making product characterization and structure-function relationships difficult to predict.[4]

The starting material is usually a stroma free-Hb (SFH), or stroma poor Hb, obtained after red cells lysis followed by filtration and chromatographic procedures, which will invariably result in a mixture of Hb and other red cell proteins in solution before chemical modifications.[5] Anionic and cationic chromatographic procedures have been used to produce, in some cases, an extremely purified human Hb known as HbA_0 that has demonstrated purity of approximately 99%. This Hb has been used to produce a polymeric form of HbA_0.[6]

Chemical modifications in general aims at stabilizing Hb in tetrameric (as found within red blood cells [RBCs]), or the polymeric form using SFH or the highly purified HbA_0 to primarily increase intravascular retention and the prevention of renal filtration by smaller, molecular-size fractions of the protein. Hb tetramer or stabilized tetramer has been successfully expressed in host systems, such a bacteria using recombinant technology.[7] The term blood substitutes has been loosely and inaccurately used to describe these therapeutics as these proteins are not capable of performing other functions of blood, such as transport, defense, and protection, rather they are being primarily used as volume replacement and as oxygen bridging agents.

Fig. 1 lists some of the most commonly used HBOCs and key chemical features, including molecular size distribution and the type and nature of the chemical reagents used. This figure also summarizes some physiochemical properties together with their oxygen and oxidation chemistries.

Characterization of complex chemical or recombinant modifications imparted on Hb has been the focus of the author's laboratory. These molecular modifications are essential for the use of Hb as an oxygen carrier in a cell-free environment. However, these typical approaches to manufacturing HBOCs can induce random non-site specific modifications to critical regions of the protein and may result in

Hemoglobin (Sponsor)	Molecular Size (kDa)	% tetramer (Modifying reagent)	Redox potential $E_{1/2}$	Autoxidation k (h^{-1})	P_{50} mmHg/ (n_{50})	General Structure(s)
HbA$_0$	64	100	82.9	0.011	12 (2.6)	
DCLHb (Baxter)	64-70	95 (Bis-(3,5-dibromosalicyl) fumarate)	124.7	0.024	30 (2.3)	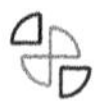
Hemopure (Biopure)	87 - 502	3-4% (Glutaraldehyde)	100.5	0.036	49 (1.4)	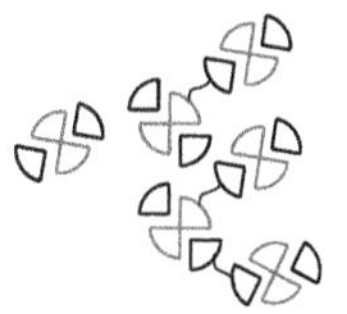
HbDex	300 (64 to > 600)	0 (Dextran)	93.6	0.042	26 (1.3)	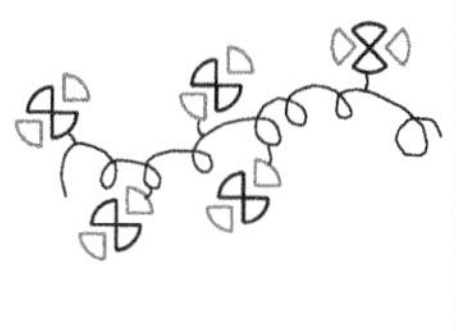
Hemolink (Hemosol)	32 to > 600 (5% dimer / un-stabilized tetramer)	32.7 (Open ring trisaccharide ; O-raffinose)	96.8	0.039	51 (1.0)	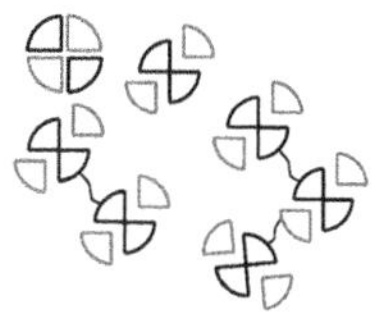
Oxyglobin (Hemopure)	87- 502	37.2 (Glutaraldehyde)	106.1	0.036	45 (1.3)	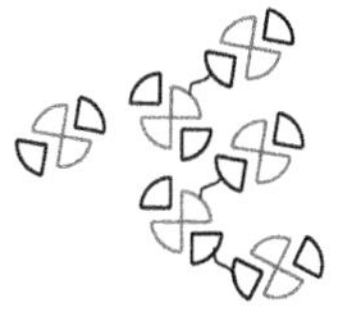

Fig. 1. Structural and some biophysical characteristics of commonly used HBOCs. Molecular sizes are based on size-exclusion chromatography coupled with multi-angle laser light scattering, or published studies where indicated.[2] Gray wedges (α globin), black wedges (β globin). *Abbreviations:* Redox potential ($E_{1/2}$), midpoint redox potential (a measure of susceptibility of Hb toward oxidation); Oxygen affinity (P_{50}), oxygen half saturation of Hb (P_{50}s for some HBOCs [eg Oxyglobin, Hemopure, and Hemolink]) reported in **Fig. 1**, were recalculated using Adair equations to allow for the fact that their OECs are not fully saturated at $PO_2 = 100$ mmHg (see **Fig. 2**); Cooperativity (n_{50}), refers to the communication between the different heme centers within Hb; Autoxidation rate (k [h^{-1}]), the rate of oxidation of the ferrous iron of Hb to the ferric nonfunctional form. (*DCLHb was a kind gift from the US army; Hemopure, Oxyglobin and Hemolink were kind gifts from Biopure and Hemosol respectively. HbDex was a kind gift from Dr. Patrick Menu of University of Henri Poincare-Nancy, France.*)

destabilization of the Hb molecule. One particular HBOC, *O*-raffinose polymerized Hb (*O*-R-polyHbA$_0$) (Hemolink), which has been in clinical development for some time can be used as an example to illustrate this point. Like other products, this particular HBOC produces toxicity in the heart and brain.[2] We have investigated the molecular basis for this protein's unusual functional profile and how this may have potentially contributed to these toxicologic events.

O-R-polyHbA$_0$ is an intra-and intermolecularly cross-linked derivative of deoxygenated human HbAo, using the cross-linking reagent, the oxidized trisaccharide, O-raffinose. When compared with its native protein (HbA$_0$), O-R-polyHbA$_0$ was found to be locked in the T (tense) (deoxy) quaternary conformation with a lower oxygen (O$_2$) affinity, a reduced Bohr effect (50% of HbA$_0$), no measurable cooperativity ($n = 1$), and a diminished response to inositol hexaphosphate, an allosteric modifier of Hb function. Other properties consistent with a T-like conformation are reduced accessibility of the β93Cys thiol group of O-R-polyHbA$_0$.[8]

The structural and functional abnormalities documented earlier may have contributed to the unusual clinical adverse events profile of O-R-polyHbA$_0$. We have therefore reasoned that there may exist some structural constraints on the molecule, the origin of which may lie within one or more fractions of this heterogeneous polymeric Hb. Using size exclusion chromatography, we separated the heterogeneous O-R-poly HbA$_0$ mixture of polymers into six distinct fractions with a molecular weight distribution ranging from 64 to approximately 600 kDa. Oxygen equilibrium and kinetics binding parameters of all fractions were the same, reflecting a lack of heterogeneity in ligand binding properties among O-R-polyHbAo species. Peptide analysis of the enzymatically digested Hb derivative and its isolated fractions were performed using liquid chromatography tandem mass spectrometry (LCMS/MS). Proposed sites of intramolecular cross-linking (βLys82, βLys82 and βVal1) by the manufacturer were found to be unaltered and abundant in the sequence ID of O-R-polyHbA$_0$. Intermolecular cross-linking with O-raffinose surprisingly resulted instead in extensive amino acid modification of key amino, such as β93Cys and β104Cys residues. These findings, combined with the documented functional and oxidative peculiarities, allowed us to provide some molecular basis for the reported adverse reactions upon infusion of O-R-polyHbA$_0$.[9] Additionally, mass spectrometry, particularly peptide sequencing by LC/MS/MS, has allowed us for the first time to identify the patterns of amino acid modifications on the proteins and has enabled us to determine the nature and extent of these modifications on the molecular integrity of HBOCs.

Armed with these powerful tools our group evaluated several HBOCs as models for site-specific modification with the intent to provide further guidance on the appropriate characterization of these products.[9–11]

POTENCY AND BIOLOGIC ACTIVITY OF HEMOGLOBIN-BASED OXYGEN CARRIERS

One of the critical questions that occupied industrial, academic, and regulatory scientists is whether HBOCs deliver sufficient oxygen to tissues. Several invasive and noninvasive techniques were used to monitor oxygen delivery by HBOCs, which resulted in conflicting and unsatisfactory data in animals and in humans.

Techniques that generate a set of oxygen equilibrium curves (OECs) are the most commonly used bioassays in vitro that reflect HBOCs oxygen-binding characteristics under well-controlled experimental conditions, such as temperature, pH, and oxygen tension. A host of important biochemical attributes can be derived from these bioassays, such as oxygen-binding equilibrium constants; allosteric modulations and sensitivities; and cooperativity, a term used to describe the relationship between the different heme centers within the Hb molecule. **Fig. 2** shows typical oxygen equilibrium curves for several HBOCs contrasted with that of a fresh RBC and an isolated purified Hb (HbA$_0$). It is evident that the position and shape of these OECs are different; some retained their classical sigmoidal shape, whereas others lack such an important

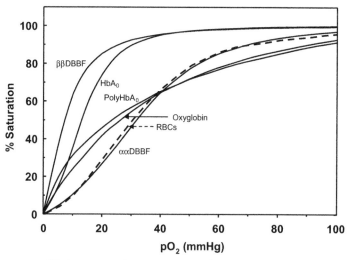

Fig. 2. Oxygen equilibrium curves for some commonly used HBOCs compared with that of HbA_0 and fresh red blood cells. Oxygen affinity (p50) values derived from these OECs for some HBOCs are reported in **Fig. 1**.

cooperative behavior, are either left or right shifted, and some curves do not even saturate at higher oxygen tension (ie, $PO_2 = 100$ mmHg). This variability complicates interpretations of the in vitro potency assessment let alone the predictive value of their physiologic performance. The debate within the community on whether oxygen-binding properties should match that of the RBCs (ie, low oxygen affinity [large $P_{50} =$ oxygen half saturation] or high oxygen affinity [small P_{50}]) is still raging with no animal or human data available to convincingly support either arguments.[12]

We were first to recognize that the transcriptional factor, hypoxia-inducible factor (HIF-1α), can be used as a valuable oxygen sensor or a preclinical biomarker of tissue oxygenation.[13] As the master regulator of oxygen homeostasis, HIF-1α has been characterized for its important functional role for mammals in the transcriptional regulation of major pathway genes that mediate the adaptive responses to hypoxia and oxidative stress, such as anemia and high altitude. We have previously documented in culture media of bovine aortic endothelia cells, and more recently in human kidney cells (HK293), a clear correlation between oxygen carrying (P_{50}) redox states of HBOCs and the expression of HIF-1α, and that this relationship can be refined further as a reliable index of HBOCs functionality and toxicity under a variety of controlled, experimental conditions.[13]

Subsequently, we showed in rats and guinea pigs, as models of HBOC exchange transfusion for blood, that a crosstalk can be established between the infused HBOC oxygen carrier and HIF oxygen sensor.[14] We have recently documented for the first time that erythropoietic (EPO), glycolytic (ENO-1,-2), including a mitochondrial respiratory (eg, cytochrome oxidases, COX4-nb) pathways had increased in response to acute hemodilution with non-oxygen carrier, hetastarch. EPO is the principal hormone that mediates hematopoietic responses to hypoxia and is the best characterized HIF-1α –regulated mammalian gene. These responses were suppressed for the first 4 to 6 hours by allosterically stabilized HBOC, and these events can be correlated well with the oxygen carrying capacity (P_{50}) of Hb and its iron heme oxidative state.[15]

This discovery opened the door for regulating the hypoxic acclimatization state through the engineering or modification of Hb or RBCs. Concurrently, HIF genetic machinery can also be directly influenced by small molecule drugs that can target HIF enzymatic degradation pathways. It may, therefore, pave the way for a new paradigm in blood substitute research in which oxygen transport and oxygen sensing mechanisms can be manipulated to produce an affective oxygen transporting vesicle under a variety of physiologic and pathologic conditions.

TOXICITY OF HEMOGLOBIN-BASED OXYGEN CARRIERS

Progress in the development of HBOCs as viable therapeutic agents has been painfully slow and was hampered by several unexplained toxicities that have been challenging to industrial/research and regulatory communities. Reviewing published literature on the toxicities of HBOCs revealed several documented preclinical and clinical toxicities that have a common biochemical origin.[16] These events appear to emanate from, and are driven by, the heme prosthetic group of Hb. A clear example is the reaction between HBOCs and NO, an important signaling and vasodilator diatomic gas produced by the vascular system. The reaction is primarily with the heme group, which can be completed within a few seconds with a profound consequence (ie, blood vessel constriction and elevation in systematic and pulmonary blood pressures [approximate mean arterial blood pressure changes ranges bewteen15–30 mmHg]). However, blood pressure elevations seen in animals and humans appear to follow a predictable path that can return to normal within two hours.

Several strategies that focused on controlling hemodynamic imbalances after infusion of HBOCs using NO donors or the inhibition of NO synthetic pathways seemed to have blunted these responses, but with little or no long-term tangible effects on organ toxicities. Some of the most imaginative and short-term strategies to control blood-pressure elevation, including the transformation of the Hb molecule into an NO carrier (S-nitosylation of cysteine residue)[17] or enzymatically transforming Hb in the presence of nitrite into a source for NO (nitrite reductase)[18] to be delivered to tissues on the basis of the well-known allosteric transition of Hb between the two states (oxygen and non-oxygen carrying states), have also failed to resolve long-term toxicities associated with HBOCs. Similar approaches to control pulmonary blood pressure triggered by free Hb have just been emphasized by the disappointing news from a failed clinical trial that investigated a similar NO modulating strategy in sickle cell disease (http://public.nhlbi.nih.gov/newsroom/home/GetPressRelease.aspx?id=2650).

Other adverse events that have been reported may have a direct or an indirect relationship to heme reactivities, including gastrointestinal tract side effects, pancreatic and liver enzyme elevations, cardiac involvement, proinflammatory responses, neurotoxicity, and oxidative stress.[19]

Over the last 20 years, our laboratory has focused on the contribution of heme-mediated side reactions to the overall toxicity seen with the infusion of HBOCs. Hb or HBOCs, outside the protective red cell environment, undergo uncontrollably spontaneous oxidation of the ferrous heme iron ($HbFe^{II}-O_2$) to ferric $HbFe^{III}$ (metHb) and oxidants, such as superoxide ion ($O_2^{\bullet-}$) and peroxide (H_2O_2), in contrast to intraerythrocytic Hb, which is continuously reduced back to ferrous functional form by efficient enzymatic machinery within the RBCs.

$$HbFe^{II}-O_2 \rightarrow HbFe^{III} \text{ (metHb)} + O_2^{\bullet-} \text{ (autoxidation)}$$

In the presence of oxidants, such H_2O_2, produced by Hb or by other cellular sources, such as macrophages and endothelial cells, the Hb is transformed into a highly radicalized species, known as ferryl Hb ($HbFe^{IV}$), which is a highly cytotoxic species.[20]

We, and others, have asked whether the observed in vitro oxidation reactions can predict in vivo events, and if so, do these oxidation reactions in any way compromise HBOCs safety and their ability to carry oxygen? Contrary and anecdotal experimental data were presented by others to suggest that there was a disconnect or dissociation between in vitro and in vivo oxidation rates of some modified Hb.[21] Additionally, the role of endogenous reductants or clearance mechanisms in affecting overall oxidation reactions of free Hb and their impact, if any, in the real physiology is not fully understood. In recent years, we have developed sensitive animal models that specifically address these issues and showed unequivocally that these reactions do occur in experimental animal models and that oxidative changes at the protein and the surrounding tissues can indeed be identified and quantified.[14,22]

More recently we showed in two animal models, dogs and guinea pigs, that haptoglobin can limit the toxic effects of cell-free Hb infusion. Initially, we examined the effects of glucocorticoid-mediated Hp induction in dogs. Next, we evaluated the ability of Hp administered pharmacologically to prevent Hb-induced hemodynamic responses and oxidative toxicity of the extravascular environment in guinea pigs. Data obtained from both models showed that Hb-Hp complex formation[1] attenuated the hypertensive response during Hb exposure, and[2] prevented Hb peroxidative toxicity in extravascular compartments, such as the kidney.[22] Haptoglobin has been shown by our group to site-specifically bind to Hb and to protect key amino acids from oxidation.[23] It surprisingly allows Hb to perform oxygen carrying and redox reactions with peroxide unhindered. Thus, Hp not only allows Hb to consume these harmful oxidants but it also redirects and absorbs the impacts of the harmful radicals that result from these reactions. These data clearly documented for the first time that free Hb is a toxic molecule and that therapies involving supplementation of endogenous Hb scavenger pathways can be designed to treat complications of acute and chronic hemolysis. Additionally, because the Hb-Hp complex retains its NO and oxygen-binding characteristics, it seems logical that compartmentalization of Hb, rather than short lived NO-based therapies, may be useful in countering the vasoactivity associated with free Hb in hemolytic anemias and with Hb oxygen therapeutics.

SUMMARY AND FUTURE STUDIES

Recent setbacks in using Hb-based technology to develop oxygen carriers or blood substitutes may spur new and fundamentally different approaches for the development of a new generation of HBOCs. The complex biochemical changes brought about by chemical or genetic modifications onto the Hb molecule and their physiologic impact must be fully understood in vitro and in appropriately designed animal models. More predictive animal models for the evaluation of Hb safety should be developed by focusing on animal species/models that mimic aspects of human physiology, which includes tissue compartment oxidative and anti-oxidative status that predict human physiology, and developing models of endothelial dysfunction to predict Hb disease state interactions. Additionally, state-of-the-art proteomic and genomic analysis are now available that should be employed to evaluate oxidative changes in the protein and surrounding plasma and tissue proteins/genes that can be adapted to understand and predict safety of these therapeutics. Finally, it may prove necessary to explore some of the naturally occurring anti-oxidative and clearing mechanisms of acellular Hb in some organisms that have adapted selective evolutionary pressures, as a basis for future Hb-based technology.

ACKNOWLEDGMENTS

The author wishes to acknowledge Drs P. Buehler and Y. Jia for constructing **Figs. 1** and **2** respectively and Dr Dominador Manalo for reading the manuscript.

REFERENCES

1. Winslow RM. Red cell substitutes. Semin Hematol 2007;44:51–9.
2. Silverman TA, Weiskopf RB. Hemoglobin-based oxygen carriers. current status and future direction. Anesthesiology 2009;111:946–63.
3. Alayash AI. Oxygen therapeutics: can we tame haemoglobin? Nat Rev Drug Discov 2004;3:152–9.
4. Buehler PW, Vallelian F, Mikolajczyk MG, et al. Structural stabilization in tetrameric or polymeric hemoglobin determines its interaction with endogenous antioxidant scavenger pathways. Antioxid Redox Signal 2008;10:1449–62.
5. Privalle C, Talarico T, Keng T, et al. Pyridoxalated hemoglobin polyoxyethylene: a nitric oxide scavenger with antioxidant activity for the treatment of nitric oxide-induced shock. Free Radic Biol Med 2000;28:1507–17.
6. Adamson JG, Moore C. Hemolink, an O-raffinose crosslinked hemoglobin based oxygen carrier. In: Change TMS, editor. Blood substitutes: principles, methods, products and clinical trials. Basel (Switzerland): Karger; 1998. p. 62–79.
7. Looker D, Abbott-Brown D, Cozart P, et al. human recombinant haemoglobin designed for use as a blood substitute. Nature 1992;356:258–60.
8. Jia Y, Ramasamy S, Wood F, et al. Crosslinking with O-raffinose lowers oxygen affinity and stabilizes haemoglobin in a non0-cooperative T-state. Biochem J 2004;384:367–75.
9. Boykins RA, Buehler PW, Jia Y, et al. O-raffinose cross-linked hemoglobin lacks site specific chemistry in the central cavity: structural and functional consequences of beta93cys modification proteins, structure, function and informatics. Proteins 2005;59:840–55.
10. Buehler PW, Boykins RA, Jia Y, et al. Structural and functional characterization of glutaraldehyde polymerized bovine hemoglobin and its isolated fractions. Anal Chem 2005;77:3466–78.
11. Buehler PW, Boykins RA, Norris S, et al. Chemical characterization of diaspirin cross-linked hemoglobin polymerized with ploy (ethylene glycol). Anal Chem 2006;78:4634–41.
12. Vandergrift KD, Winslow RM. Hemopsan: design, principles for a new class of oxygen therapeutics. Artif Organs 2009;33:133–8.
13. Yeh LH, Alayash AI. Effects of cell-free hemoglobin on hypoxia inducible factor (HIF-1alpha) and heme oxygenase (HO-1) expression in endothelial cells subjected to hypoxia. Antioxid Redox Signal 2004;6:944–53.
14. Buehler PW, D'Agnillo F, Hoffman V, et al. Effects of endogenous ascorbate on oxidation, oxygenation and toxicokinetics of cell-free modified hemoglobin after exchange transfusion in rats and guinea pigs. J Pharmacol Exp Ther 2007;323:49–60.
15. Manalo DJ, Buehler PW, Baek JH, et al. Acellular haemoglobin attenuates hypoxia-inducible factor-1alpha (HIF-1alpha) and its target genes in haemodiluted rats. Biochem J 2008;414:461–9.
16. Winslow RM. Current status of oxygen carries ('blood substitutes'): 2006. Vox Sang 2006;91:102–10.
17. Jia L, Bonaventura C, Bonaventura J, et al. S.nitrosohaemoglobin: a dynamic activity of blood involved in vascular control. Nature 1996;380:221–6.

18. Cosby K, Partove KS, Crawford JH, et al. Nitrite reduction to nitric oxide by deoxyhemoglobin vasodilates the human circulation. Nat Med 2003;9:1498–505.

19. Mackenzie CF, Bucci C. Artificial oxygen carriers for trauma: myth or reality. Hosp Med 2004;65:562–8.

20. D'Agnillo F, Alayash AI. Redox cycling of diaspirin cross-linked hemoglobin induces G2/M arrest and apoptosis in cultured endothelial cells. Blood 2001; 98:3315–23.

21. Vandergrift KD, Malavalli A, Minn C, et al. Oxidation and haem loss kinetics of Poly(ethylene glycol)-conjugated (MP4): dissociation between in vitro and in vivo oxidation rates. Biochem J 2006;399:463–71.

22. Boretti FS, Buehler PW, D'Agnillo, et al. Sequestration of extracellular hemoglobin within haptoglobin complex decrease it hypertensive and oxidative effects in dogs and guinea pigs. J Clin Invest 2009;119:2271–80.

23. Buehler PW, Abraham B, Vallelian F, et al. Haptoglobin preserves the CD163 hemoglobin scavenger pathway by shielding hemoglobin from peroxidative modification. Blood 2009;113:2578–86.

From Stem Cell to Red Blood Cells In Vitro: "The 12 Labors of Hercules"

Luc Douay, MD, PhD

KEYWORDS

- Artificial blood • Stem cells • Hemoglobin
- Transfusion medicine

In the context of the constant difficulty of obtaining supplies of blood products, the interest of disposing of complementary sources of red blood cells (RBCs) for transfusion is evident. The development of chemical or natural molecules that would replace hemoglobin is proving difficult. Artificial blood is still unattainable. Hence, instead of replacing what is made by nature, why not copy it? For these reasons, attempting to generate red blood cells in the laboratory makes sense. This article describes the research in progress that will permit the large-scale production of human red blood cells from hematopoietic stem cells. It also discusses the state of the art of this concept, suggests the obstacles to be overcome to pass from the laboratory model to clinical practice, and analyzes the possible indications in the medium and long term. The potential interest of pluripotent stem cells as an unlimited source of RBCs is considered. If it succeeds, this new approach could mark a considerable advance in the field of transfusion.

WHY SEARCH FOR NEW SOURCES OF RBCS?
Demographic Demands for Transfusion Medicine

The demographic evolution predicted in the United States[1] indicates an important increase in the proportion of people over 60 years of age, estimated to be about 18% in 2000, 20% in 2010, 25% in 2030, and 26% in 2050. An even more rapid aging of the population is anticipated in France,[2] where the percentage of persons over 60 years will go from 21% in 2004 to 23% in 2010, 29% in 2030, and 32% in 2050. This aging of the population will have two important consequences for blood transfusion. On the one hand, it will lead to a considerable increase in malignant hematologic conditions; for example, acute myeloblastic leukemias, chronic myeloid leukemias,

UMR_S938, Proliferation and differentiation of stem cells, INSERM, UPMC Univ Paris 06, Etablissement Français du Sang Ile de France, F-94200, Ivry-sur-Seine, France
E-mail address: luc.douay@trs.aphp.fr

Clin Lab Med 30 (2010) 391–403
doi:10.1016/j.cll.2010.02.003   labmed.theclinics.com
0272-2712/10/$ – see front matter © 2010 Elsevier Inc. All rights reserved.

and non-Hodgkin's lymphomas, the frequency of which increases with age[3] and which have important requirements for transfusion. Hence, on the same basis as before and assuming that the incidence of these conditions as a function of age remains stable, one can predict that their global incidence will increase by about 60% in France and 100% in the United States from now to 2050. On the other hand, the number of persons of an age to give blood will rise much more slowly than will the need for blood components. Still considering the demographic projections established for the United States and France, one may deduce that the population of an age to give blood will increase by only 6% in France and 35% in the United States from now to 2050, whereas the general population will grow by 16% and 49% respectively. Therefore, whether we wish it or not, it will be mandatory to find alternatives to conventional transfusion practices.

The Challenge of Oxygen Carrier Substitutes

The idea of artificial blood, universal and safe, has been in circulation for more than 50 years. There is no hope, even in the long term, of replacing the white cells that defend us against infections or the platelets that initiate blood coagulation in the event of bleeding. The dream of artificial blood has to be limited to the red cells—primordial cells having essentially only one function, to transport oxygen and deliver it to all the tissues of the body. This vital function is ensured by a special pigment, hemoglobin. Hence, when one speaks of artificial blood, one is simply talking about replacing this hemoglobin.

Can we replace such a refined cellular mode such as the RBC? At first sight, that blood cell might seem extremely uninteresting, a simple bag which has lost the vital elements, like its nucleus. It is, in reality, a cell that has pushed its specialization, oxygen transport, to the point of eliminating all that is not useful.

However, this cell knows how to be unique. At its surface, there exist more than thirty blood-group families, which prohibit the transfusion of any indiscriminant type of RBC to any indiscriminant receiver. By liberating hemoglobin from this bag or replacing it with a totally synthetic molecule, while still conserving its oxygen transport capacity, one would attain the objective of an artificial blood. A recent meta-analysis recently reported a 30% increased risk of myocardial infarction in patients who received hemoglobin substitutes.[4]

One can turn to artificial oxygen transporters such as the perfluorocarbon molecules, but these synthetic molecules are unstable in the blood stream. Hence, they cannot carry out their role of oxygenation for very long—24 to 48 hours at the most—and they can in no way provide long-term transfusion support for a patient who lacks RBCs.

Nothing has yet led to a concrete therapeutic application. Much time has gone by. It is now several decades that we have been looking for a substitute for RBCs. In vain! Nature is not so easy to replace.

RBCs from Stem Cells

If one cannot replace nature, why not "simply" copy her? We indeed have sufficient knowledge of the biology of hematopoietic stem cells (HSC) to hope to generate human RBCs in the laboratory. One may reasonably predict that it will soon be possible to produce enough to transfuse "cultured" red blood cells (cRBC).[5]

HSCs represent 1 cell in 10,000 in the bone marrow. In close contact with the medullar microenvironment, they proliferate and differentiate according to a well-defined hierarchy to give rise to the different cell lines of the blood.[6] We have known since the 1980s that HSC are very numerous in umbilical cord blood.[7] One can also make them pass from the bone marrow to the blood by injecting specific growth factors, which facilitates their collection. The medullar microenvironment is composed of different cells, grouped under the generic name of stromal cells. These cells secrete soluble factors which regulate the production of HSC and facilitate their interactions.[8,9]

This fundamental knowledge of hematopoiesis has enabled us to improve the practice of bone marrow grafting and to widen the concept to the grafting of HSC from peripheral blood or umbilical cord blood. We have been trying for about 10 years to improve the grafting of HSC by increasing the numbers of these cells in the grafts. One study focused on ex vivo expansion.[10] While working on this problem, it was tempting to force the cells to differentiate specifically to the RBC line, known as the erythroid line. This cell line nevertheless has an essential particularity: at the end of its maturation in the bone marrow, the erythroid cell expels its nucleus before entering the blood stream. This is the birth of the RBC, the only cell of the body to have a long life span, 120 days, despite the absence of a nucleus. In this context, an attempt to generate erythroid cells in vitro through amplification of stem cells makes good sense.

We can let our scientific imagination run wild for an instant and dream of the ideal transfusion of tomorrow: an automated production of universal RBC from an infinite source of HSC, replacing the present system based on volunteer donors. A so-called blood-farming program would aim at developing new technologies to enable the in vitro production of RBCs that are pure, readily available, and free of storage lesions. The ultimate goal of such a program would be the development of an automated cell culture and packaging system capable of generating transfusable amounts of universal donor (type O/Rh negative) RBC using human stem cells as the starting material. The RBC produced by the system would be the functional equivalent of donor-derived RBC and induce no greater responses than normal donor-derived RBC. The result would be an automated culture system that would (1) maintain a self-renewing progenitor cell population, (2) support the differentiation, separation, and packaging of transfusable RBC, and (3) be ready for submission to worldwide regulation agencies for all applicable device and transfusable cell product approvals.

To achieve these goals, revolutionary advances in research areas such as the control of progenitor cell expansion or differentiation and the development of automated bioreactors capable of automated cell manipulation and purification would be necessary. Just an impossible dream? Let us analyze the obstacles to be overcome—something like the twelve labors of Hercules.

Overcoming these obstacles means creating in vitro the experimental conditions satisfying three requirements: stimulation of the proliferation of primitive HSC, induction of their exclusive commitment to the erythroid line, and completion of their terminal maturation to the stage of enucleated cells.

LABOR #1: PROLIFERATION AND ERYTHROID COMMITMENT

Neildez-Nguyen and colleagues[11] initially described a protocol for the expansion of HSC derived from cord blood in a well-defined medium without stroma, based on the sequential addition of growth factors. Starting from CD34+ cells, this protocol allowed the massive production (amplification up to 200,000 times) of pure erythroid precursors (up to 99%) containing fetal hemoglobin (HbF). Contrary to what happens under these ex vivo conditions in the presence of growth factors alone, when such progenitors or precursors are injected into NOD-SCID mice, they were capable of continuing to proliferate in vivo and of differentiating within 4 days to the terminal stage of enucleated cells producing adult hemoglobin.

The first step is overcome since we are able to induce an exclusive erythroid differentiation with a level of amplification compatible with transfusion medicine requirements. That first observation demonstrates that if a large level of expansion could be reached in vitro, full differentiation only occurred in vivo pointing to a major role of the microenvironment in terminal erythroid differentiation.

LABOR #2: PROLIFERATION AND TERMINAL MATURATION

The need for an in vitro reconstitution of the bone marrow microenvironment became obvious. On the basis of these data, investigators subsequently modified the protocol to obtain the expansion and differentiation of CD34+ cells derived from blood, bone marrow, or cord blood in three steps[12]: (1) in a liquid medium, involving cell proliferation and induction of erythroid differentiation in the presence of stem cell factor, interleukin-3, and erythropoietin (Epo); (2) based on a model reconstitution of the microenvironment (murine stromal cell line MS5), in the presence of Epo alone; (3) in the presence of the stromal cells alone, without any growth factors. This cell culture system in a well-defined medium without serum reproduces ex vivo the microenvironment existing in vivo (**Fig. 1**).

Using this protocol, we obtain, after 15, days a plateau of the mean amplification of CD34+ cells of 20,000-fold for cells from bone marrow or peripheral blood, 30,000-fold for cells obtained by leukapheresis after mobilization with G-CSF, and 200,000-fold for cells derived from cord blood. A total commitment to the erythroid lineage is morphologically evident after 8 days. Differentiation of the reticulocytes into mature RBCs continues from day 15 to day 18, as shown by the further disappearance of nuclei, progressive loss of transferrin receptor CD71 expression, and staining with laser dye styryl (LDS). At this stage, 90% to 100% of the cells are enucleated. These erythrocytes display characteristics close to those of native RBCs (volume and haemoglobin content).

On an immunologic basis, cRBCs express at their surface the very same blood group antigens compared with native cells (**Fig. 2**). We further tested more than 25 blood-group antigen families without noting any difference.

LABOR # 3: MATURATION AND CONSERVATION OF RETICULOCYTES

The population generated in vitro is mainly composed of reticulocytes. The main feature is that the experimental conditions are not favorable to maturation up to final

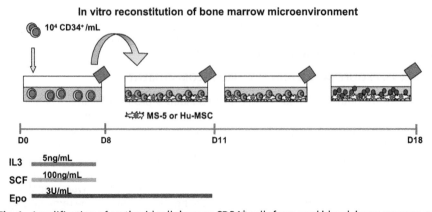

In vitro reconstitution of bone marrow microenvironment

Fig. 1. Amplification of erythroid cells human CD34+ cells from cord blood, bone marrow, or peripheral blood are cultured in a liquid medium on a layer of stromal cells of murine origin (MS5) according to a three-phase protocol.

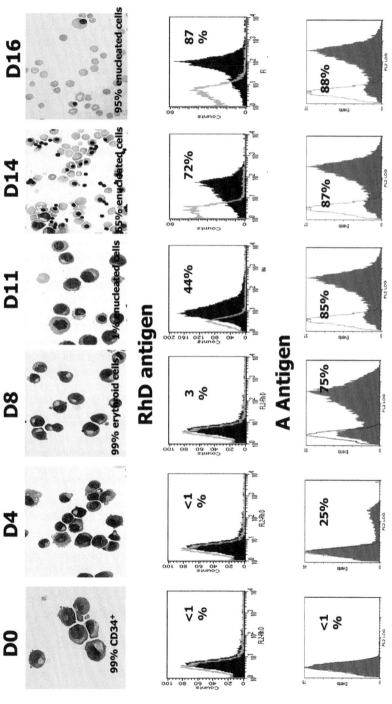

Fig. 2. Blood group antigen expression along the culture.

RBCs. Once produced, reticulocytes have to be transferred into a defined medium unless they hemolyze. That point is crucial for further clinical use if full maturation is required. Fortunately, as described below, in vivo maturation occurs.

The conservation of cRBCs is possible up to at least 30 days in vitro. It is, however, mandatory to design conditions dedicated to the status of reticulocytes, that is, different from the ones commonly used for native RBCs (eg, Sagmanitol).

LABOR #4: TERMINAL DIFFERENTIATION INTO ADULT AND FUNCTIONAL HEMOGLOBIN

The reticulocytes and cRBCs generated ex vivo have to be functionally equivalent to donor-derived RBC. That is the case because:

1. They have glucose-6-phosphate dehydrogenase and pyruvate kinase levels in keeping with the properties of a young homogenous RBC population. This indicates that they are capable of reducing glutathione and maintaining ATP levels and, therefore, have a normal level of 2, 3-diphosphoglycerate.
2. Their deformability, as evaluated by ektacytometry, is comparable to that of native erythrocytes.
3. The functionality of the hemoglobin present in cRBC is assessed by ligand-binding kinetics after flash photolysis. The bimolecular kinetics after photodissociation of CO provides a sensitive test of hemoglobin function. On varying the energy of the photolysis pulse, two phases are observed which correspond to the two hemoglobin conformations (R and T states). The kinetics are thus biphasic, reflecting the two allosteric forms.
4. Like native hemoglobin, cRBC hemoglobin is able to fix and release oxygen. Oxygen equilibrium measurements confirm the observed affinity and cooperativity. The log (P50) value is 1.2 for cRBC hemoglobin as compared with 1.3 for control RBC hemoglobin and the Hill coefficients are identical (N50 of 2.28 vs 2.29). The kinetic and equilibrium data, therefore, indicate ligand-binding properties in very close agreement with control values. Methemoglobin is not detected, which shows that cRBC are enzymatically capable of reversing hemoglobin oxidation.

Interestingly, starting from BM or LK CD34+, the in vitro generated RBCs contained a great majority of adult hemoglobin. On the contrary, starting from cord blood CD34+ cells, they contained a great majority of HbF, probably secondary to the proliferating status of these various sources.

LABOR #5: SIMPLIFICATION OF THE PROCEDURE TO AVOID MICROENVIRONMENT RECONSTITUTION

In an attempt to simplify the culture process, Miharada and colleagues[13] developed a stroma-free protocol for ex vivo production of enucleated RBCs. Although they successfully demonstrated that stromal elements were not an absolute requirement for enucleation, expansion was only 700,000-fold with a degree of enucleation of 77.5% compared with the 98% previously reported by Giarratana and colleagues.[12] These data were in accordance with the author's observation that, although contact between stromal cells and erythroid cells is useful for erythroid proliferation, it is not mandatory for enucleation. Indeed, in this system, elimination of the direct contact between MS-5 cells and erythroid cells by a 0.45 μm transwell did not abrogate all enucleation. Interestingly, stromal cells are highly involved in the nuclei phagocytosis. These results are strong arguments for the fact that stromal cells produce soluble factors permitting erythroblast maturation up to enucleation.

The key success, therefore, relies on designing a define culture medium that mimics the microenvironment but avoiding the complexity of a coculture system. It was shown that reticulocytes generated in vitro in the presence of a defined culture medium and three growth factors (stem cell factor, interleukin-3, and Epo), but in the absence of coculture with stromal cells, have all the necessary functional characteristics in terms of enzymatic content, membrane deformability, and the capacity of hemoglobin to fix and release oxygen.

Attempts to improve the system have been looked for. For instance, Fujimi and colleagues[14] proposed to cultivate cord blood CD34+ cells on a telomerase gene transduced (hTERT) human stromal cell line, followed by a period of monoculture, subsequently succeeded by a period in coculture with macrophages derived from parallel cocultures of CD34+ cells (from a different donor) on hTERT stromal cells in the presence of macrophage colony stimulating factor and granulocyte colony stimulating factor. In a final phase, enucleation was achieved as described by Miharada and colleagues.[13] Given that the yield per umbilical cord blood donation was no greater than that achieved previously,[12] the added complexity and associated costs of this method would be difficult to justify in a manufacturing environment.

LABOR #6: IN VIVO LIFESPAN STUDY

After intraperitoneal infusion into NOD-SCID mice, CFSE-labeled cRBC and reticulocytes obtained by apheresis persist in the circulation to the same extent as CFSE-labeled native RBC: CFSE+ cells are detected for 3 days in both groups of transfused animals. In vivo, the transfused reticulocytes fully mature into RBC as shown by the appearance of CFSE+/LDS- cells. Over 90% of the CFSE+ cells are mature RBCs by day 3. The next step will be to demonstrate in vivo in humans that cRBC have a normal lifespan of close to 120 days, work which is currently in progress.

Of major interest for cRBC transfusion is the fact that it should enable the infusion of a cell population homogeneous in age with a life span close to 120 days compared with the mean half-life of 28 days of heterogeneous normal donor RBCs. This minimizes the number of transfusions required by serially transfused patients, reducing the potential of iron overload or the development of alloimmunization.

LABOR #7: QUANTITATIVE ASPECT—2000×10^9 RBCS OR 10^9 PER PACKED-RBC UNIT

If the objective is to generate RBCs from HSC for the purpose of transfusion, we immediately face the problem of the quantity of cells to be produced: one unit of conventional packed RBC contains more or less 2000 billions of cells! The challenge is therefore to exploit at the maximum the proliferation or differentiation capacity of HSC up to exhaustion to reach terminal maturation as much as possible.

In the author's experience, the best source for that purpose clearly is cord blood derived HSC. They generate 5- to 10-fold more RBCs than HSC derived from peripheral blood, in relation with an increased proliferating capacity while the enucleation capacity is similar.

In experimental conditions, in presence of a defined culture medium in a stroma-free system, combining a first phase of HSC amplification followed by a second phase of erythroid differentiation, enable generation of 4 to 22 million RBC from one cord blood CD34+ cell. Extrapolating these data to an average cord blood containing 5 million CD34+ cells, that is the equivalent of 10 to 50 packed RBC units, which could be produced in vitro from only one cord blood unit!

The benchmark is reached. Now the challenge is the industrial production.

LABOR #8: SPECIFIC INDICATIONS FOR AUTOLOGOUS SUPPORT

One potentially major indication of cRBCs concerns patients with myelodysplastic syndrome. They indeed require long-term RBC transfusion support, with major alloimmunization and infectious risks. In that situation, they would draw benefit from autologous cRBCs generated from their own peripheral hematopoietic progenitor cells. One of the key question deals with the capacity of these erythroid precursors to reach terminal maturation, that is, enucleation, because myelodysplastic syndrome is classically reported as a qualitative rather than quantitative erythroid defect. Using the model of in vitro generation of mature RBC from human HSC to the 5q(del) syndrome, it is shown that (1) the erythroid commitment of the pathologic clones is not altered, (2) their terminal differentiation capacity is preserved since they can achieve final erythroid maturation up to the stage of enucleation, and (3) the drop in RBC production is secondary to the decrease in the pool of erythroid progenitor cells and the alteration of their proliferative capacity.[15] These data open the way to that indication pending our capacity to dramatically increase cell proliferation.

Patients with sickle cell disease are the second major candidates. A high level of HbF within the sickle RBCs is correlated with a decrease of sickling. Therefore, an autologous cRBC product engineered to have a high level of HbF could be designed. Work is in progress to evaluate the feasibility and interest of this approach based on functional properties: increase in the level of HbF, diminution of sickle cell formation, diminution of adherence, and modification of the metabolomic profile. Preliminary results for RBC derived from peripheral CD34+ cells of homozygous patients support this hypothesis: tripling the level of HbF in sickle RBC reduced sickle cell formation by one-half.

LABOR #9: UNIVERSAL RBCS

This culture system offers a new approach to the search for "universal" cRBCs, that is, RBCs lacking membrane expression of the two principal blood group systems, ABO and RHD. It is no longer a question of trying to eliminate the surface antigens once they have formed, but a matter of preventing their synthesis before the cRBCs reach maturity. The blood group antigens ABO and RH, which are not expressed on HSCs, are already present on erythroblast precursors. Two approaches may be envisioned:

1. Inhibition of gene expression in CD34+ human HSCs through use of interfering RNA (siRNA). This technique enables posttranscription inhibition of a gene in a sequence-specific manner by employing doubled stranded RNA to provoke degradation of the homologous messenger RNA. Such inhibition of the expression of genes has been partially achieved using antisense oligonucleotides or ribozymes, but the approach is limited by the instability of the molecules introduced.
2. Biochemical intracellular inhibition of the glycosyltransferases specific for the antigens A and B.

Whatever the mechanism, this inhibition has to be initiated at the stage of CD34+ HSCs and continued to that of cRBCs. The methods of this approach can in fact avoid the side effects inherent to the procedures of antigen stripping or antigen masking currently being tested.

A new laboratory tool: focusing on the Kidd blood group system that relies on expression of hUT-B1 glycoprotein under the Jka or Jkb antigenic configurations, Bagnis and colleagues[16] demonstrated that hematopoietic progenitors could be genetically modified to exhibit a chosen Kidd phenotype.

Beyond production of atypical Kidd phenotypes, this genetic strategy could allow generation of rare blood phenotypes from hematopoietic stem cells regardless of initial donor phenotype. Potential applications for genetically modified blood include production of control samples for immunohematologic testing and for resolution of antibody detection in multiple transfused patients.

Finally, the simplest way to provide universal O Rh negative cRBCs would be to collect cord blood cells from donors with that specific phenotype. That represents the most common and easiest unlimited source of stem cells.

LABOR #10: UNLIMITED SOURCE OF STEM CELLS—THE PROMISES OF PLURIPOTENT STEM CELLS

As in many other therapeutic applications, human embryonic stem cells (hESCs) and related technologies, for example, induced pluripotent stem cells (iPSCs), could provide an essentially unlimited and well-characterized supply of starting material from which to manufacture RBCs. Several studies have shown that hESC cultures can be induced to undergo hematopoietic differentiation, which leads to the generation of primitive (nucleated) RBCs.[17] More recently, Lu and colleagues[18] were able to obtain 3×10^{10} primitive RBCs from a single six-well plate of hESCs, equal to an approximately 3000-fold expansion. These investigators also described the generation of mature enucleated RBCs from hESCs by a divergent process. However, a numerical expansion of only 30- to 50-fold was achieved, with an enucleation frequency of 40%. A much better understanding and reproduction of the embryonic and fetal processes leading to adult HSCs will be required before hESCs can replace HSCs as a starting material. Nevertheless, this result demonstrates that it is possible to obtain enucleated RBCs from hESC cultures.

The generation of RBCs from reprogrammed human adult stem cells, or iPSCs,[19] is to be shown yet. This would open the way to putative new developments since iPSCs could provide allogeneic as well as autologous sources of cultured RBCs. However, the same limitations exist as with hESCs concerning the amplification capacity of these cells and significant improvements in proliferative capacity will be a prerequisite to their potential use for transfusion purposes. In any case, one of the main interests of RBCs derived from hESCs or iPSCs is the very low risk of teratogenicity in the final product, since RBCs are enucleated cells easy to purify by conventional filtration. Although the underlying biology of RBC expansion and differentiation has yet to be fully elucidated, achievements over the past few years are promising. It seems likely that hESCs or iPSCs and related technologies will, in time, surpass umbilical cord blood and other donated material as a source of starting material, in many respects eliminating supply constraints.

LABOR #11: INDUSTRIAL DEVELOPMENT FOR CLINICAL APPLICATION

The ultimate and decisive challenge is to design production procedures compatible with the requirements of good manufacturing practices. A certain number of obstacles have to be overcome: (1) reduction by a factor of 100 of the quantity of medium necessary during the culture phases through use of a medical bioreactor continuously adapting the culture conditions to the cell amplification in a constant volume, (2) development of a rigorously defined culture medium containing no animal proteins, and (3) sequential addition of the cytokines by means of the bioreactor, which will increase their efficacy while reducing the quantities necessary.

If these technical developments allow us to overcome the quantitative limits, at least theoretically, the practical question of the manipulation of such culture volumes remains unresolved. Static culture methods using flasks, dishes, or gas permeable bags are not feasible. Innovative bioreactor technologies enabling more compact geometries and higher cell densities are therefore required.

The tools needed include bioreactors. Several types of bioreactor have been used to culture hematopoietic cells.[20,21] The typical approach to scale up a cell culture bioprocess is to move from a two-dimensional surface to a stirred three-dimensional tank reactor, which permits efficient mass transport even on very large scales.

Bioreactors allow control of several major parameters. First, they allow the automated monitoring and control of environmental factors such as pH, temperature, and dissolved oxygen concentration. These parameters have a significant influence on culture performance and their careful optimization is mandatory to reach clinically significant cell yields. This is notably true for hematopoietic cell culture. Control of oxygen tension[22,23] regulates both the expansion kinetics and the commitment of cultured hematopoietic cells,[14] while pH control acts similarly.[24]

The key question is how to overcome the cell density limitation inherent to static systems. Dynamic systems using membrane perfusion bioreactors will probably increase this limit by up to a factor of 100.

Although bioreactors have been successfully employed for the culture of hematopoietic cells, they have not yet been used to manufacture standard donor products such as RBCs. Due to the very large number of cells required, the existing bioreactor technologies are insufficient to meet the demands of routine RBC manufacture and new breakthroughs in related technologies will be necessary.

An automated cell culture system capable of maintaining a self-renewing progenitor population, which provides an environment for efficient erythroid differentiation and allows sorting or purification and packaging of the end product RBC in a manner directly suitable for transfusion, does not yet exist. It also has to be kept in mind that an automated culture or packaging system must operate with minimal user intervention. To achieve these aims, revolutionary advances will be necessary in areas such as the control of progenitor cell expansion or differentiation and the development of bioreactors capable of automated cell manipulation and purification.

LABOR #12: TO FIND THE MARKET

Without pretending to replace "classical" transfusion, these products could at least find indications in the context of "impossible" transfusion situations. Such situations are encountered in two circumstances: the need for rare RBC phenotypes and anti-RBC antigen poly-immunization. Moreover, certain patients are dependent for life on RBC transfusions from a very early age, such as those suffering from hemoglobinopathies, notably thalassemia, could also benefit from these products. Finally, they could be used in the case of such cRBC transfusions in intensive care.

SUMMARY: TRANSFUSION IN THE YEAR 2020

Let us imagine a possible scenario for cRBC production in 2020 as illustrated in **Fig. 3**. If this scenario becomes reality sometime during the 21st century, a simple skin biopsy could be used to generate an iPSC master-cell bank from an adult with aplastic anemia or myeloid leukemia. These cells could then be amplified and induced to differentiate into mesodermal cells and subsequently into HSCs for cRBC production. An important step toward this futuristic goal was recently achieved in a mouse model of sickle cell anemia by transplanting hematopoietic cells generated by iPSC methods after correction of the sickle cell abnormality by homologous recombination.[24]

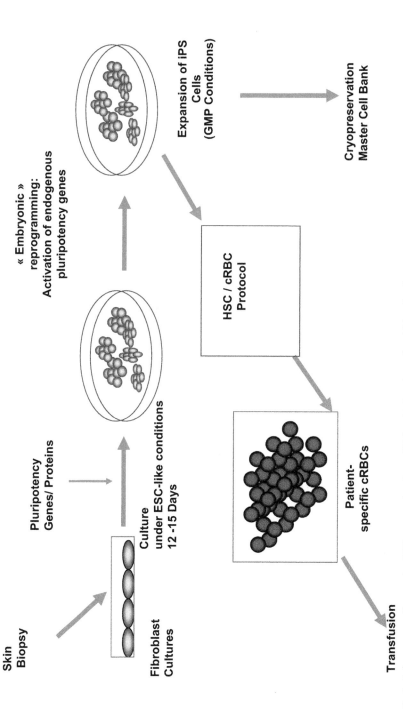

Fig. 3. Autologous or allogeneic cRBC generation from iPSCs. cRBC, cultured red blood cell; ESC, embryonic stem cell; GMP, good manufacturing practices; HSC, hematopoietic stem cells; iPS, induced pluripotent stem cells.

Although the arrival of artificial blood has been announced for a long time (more than 5 decades), we are still waiting for authentic blood substitutes. Is this an indication that in the case of cultured blood components it will not be easy to replace nature? The concept of the cultured RBC shows that it is at least possible to imitate nature. It now remains to create the technical conditions for the industrial development of cRBCs and to demonstrate the clinical and economic interest of this new blood product with simple characteristics: a concentrate of homogeneous cRBCs having a long life span, improved storage capacity, and selected phenotype, free of platelets, leukocytes, and plasma and constantly available. The path to the clinical production unit will be long, 5 to 10 years perhaps. In other words—tomorrow!

REFERENCES

1. Jc D. Population projections of the United States by age, sex, race and Hispanic origin: 1995 to 2050. Current Population Reports. Washington, DC: U.S. Bureau of the Census; 1996. p. 25.
2. Robert-Bobée I. Projections de population pour la France métropolitaine à l'horizon 2050. Paris: INSEE Première; 2006.
3. Group USCSW. United States cancer statistics: 2002 incidence and mortality. Atlanta (GA): U.S. Department of Health and Human Services, Centers of Disease Control and Prevention and National Cancer Institute; 2005.
4. Natanson C, Kern SJ, Lurie P, et al. Cell-free hemoglobin-based blood substitutes and risk of myocardial infarction and death: a meta-analysis. JAMA 2008;299: 2304.
5. Douay L, Andreu G. Ex vivo production of human red blood cells from hematopoietic stem cells: what is the future in transfusion? Transfus Med Rev 2007;21:91.
6. Ogawa M. Differentiation and proliferation of hematopoietic stem cells. Blood 1993;81:2844.
7. Lu L, Xiao M, Shen RN, et al. Enrichment, characterization, and responsiveness of single primitive CD34 human umbilical cord blood hematopoietic progenitors with high proliferative and replating potential. Blood 1993;81:41.
8. Friedenstein AJ, Deriglasova UF, Kulagina NN, et al. Precursors for fibroblasts in different populations of hematopoietic cells as detected by the in vitro colony assay method. Exp Hematol 1974;2:83.
9. Verfaillie CM. Soluble factor(s) produced by human bone marrow stroma increase cytokine-induced proliferation and maturation of primitive hematopoietic progenitors while preventing their terminal differentiation. Blood 1993;82:2045.
10. Douay L. Experimental culture conditions are critical for ex vivo expansion of hematopoietic cells. J Hematother Stem Cell Res 2001;10:341.
11. Neildez-Nguyen TM, Wajcman H, Marden MC, et al. Human erythroid cells produced ex vivo at large scale differentiate into red blood cells in vivo. Nat Biotechnol 2002;20:467.
12. Giarratana MC, Kobari L, Lapillonne H, et al. Ex vivo generation of fully mature human red blood cells from hematopoietic stem cells. Nat Biotechnol 2005;23:69.
13. Miharada K, Hiroyama T, Sudo K, et al. Efficient enucleation of erythroblasts differentiated in vitro from hematopoietic stem and progenitor cells. Nat Biotechnol 2006;24:1255.
14. Fujimi A, Matsunaga T, Kobune M, et al. Ex vivo large-scale generation of human red blood cells from cord blood CD34+ cells by co-culturing with macrophages. Int J Hematol 2008;87:339.

15. Garderet L, Kobari L, Mazurier CH, et al. A new single cell culture approach demonstrates absence of terminal erythroid differentiation alterations with preservation of enucleation capacity in myelodysplastic 5q(del) clones. Haematologica 2010;95(3):398–405.
16. Bagnis C, Chapel S, Chiaroni J, et al. A genetic strategy to control expression of human blood group antigens in red blood cells generated in vitro. Transfusion 2009;49:967.
17. Qiu C, Hanson E, Olivier E, et al. Differentiation of human embryonic stem cells into hematopoietic cells by coculture with human fetal liver cells recapitulates the globin switch that occurs early in development. Exp Hematol 2005;33:1450.
18. Lu SJ, Feng Q, Park JS, et al. Biologic properties and enucleation of red blood cells from human embryonic stem cells. Blood 2008;112:4475.
19. Takahashi K, Yamanaka S. Induction of pluripotent stem cells from mouse embryonic and adult fibroblast cultures by defined factors. Cell 2006;126:663.
20. Migliaccio AR, Whitsett C, Migliaccio G. Erythroid cells in vitro: from developmental biology to blood transfusion products. Curr Opin Hematol 2009;16:259.
21. Timmins NE, Nielsen LK. Blood cell manufacture: current methods and future challenges. Trends Biotechnol 2009;27:415.
22. Vlaski M, Lafarge X, Chevaleyre J, et al. Low oxygen concentration as a general physiologic regulator of erythropoiesis beyond the EPO-related downstream tuning and a tool for the optimization of red blood cell production ex vivo. Exp Hematol 2009;37:573.
23. McAdams TA, Miller WM, Papoutsakis ET. pH is a potent modulator of erythroid differentiation. Br J Haematol 1998;103:317.
24. Hanna J, Wernig M, Markoulaki S, et al. Treatment of sickle cell anemia mouse model with iPS cells generated from autologous skin. Science 1920;318:2007.

The Three "R"s of Blood Transfusion in 2020; Routine, Reliable and Robust

Stewart Abbot, PhD

KEYWORDS

• Blood transfusion • Stem cells • Bioreactors • Large scale

CRYSTAL BALL GAZING

Rather like evolutionary change in species, progress in many scientific fields can be characterized by protracted periods of relatively minor incremental advances punctuated by transformational events that permit a step change to a radically new process or device; blood transfusion is no different.

Although James Blundell is often credited with performing the first successful transfusion in 1818, the principles underlying successful transfusions were not adequately understood to enable widespread adoption until nearly 150 years later, following the cumulative impact of a multitude of incremental and a few transformational changes. Karl Landsteiner's observations, in the early 1900s, led to the initial classification of the A and B blood groups, and nearly half a century later the classification of Rh antigens were certainly transformational and pivotal to the modern process of routine blood transfusion.

Likewise, Richard Lewisohn's discovery in 1915 that the correct concentration of sodium citrate could be used safely to prevent coagulation and permit very short-term storage of whole blood laid the foundations for the current practices of storage and distribution. More recently, blood banking and transfusion medicine has benefited from incremental and cumulatively significant advances in the ability to detect the presence of transfusion-transmittable diseases (TTDs), which has dramatically increased the safety of blood transfusion.

Predicting the future of any scientific field is never exact, but a reasonable approximation can be made through carefully considering historical rates of change together with the cumulative impact of drivers for change and technological breakthroughs in related fields that may overcome barriers to progress. Over the past 70 years, the modern process of voluntary donation, storage, and local distribution and administration of blood and blood products has been relatively inexpensive and adequate for

Celgene Cellular Therapeutics, 7 Powderhorn Drive, Warren, NJ 07059, USA
E-mail address: sabbot@celgene.com

Clin Lab Med 30 (2010) 405–417
doi:10.1016/j.cll.2010.02.010
0272-2712/10/$ – see front matter © 2010 Published by Elsevier Inc.

labmed.theclinics.com

meeting demands. In the absence of motivation driven by unmet need (clinical or market), new processes are unlikely to evolve. Recently, however, several factors have highlighted this need for improved processes, and are likely to promote transformational change in the near future.

DRIVERS OF CHANGE

For the most part, current blood transfusion services represent an excellent example of just-in-time product procurement and distribution. These services require the careful coordination of several areas, such as advertising; centralized and field-based procurement; quality assurance and control services, including TTD testing; processing and fractionation; storage facilities; inventory analysis; distribution; and obviously clinical administration teams.

Unlike other manufacturing industries, the just-in-time-like nature of red blood cell (RBC) product procurement and use is not a direct result of desire for process efficiency and associated cost savings, but it is rather necessitated by the relatively short lifespan of RBC product in vivo (~ 120 days) and in storage (up to 42 days when stored in an U.S. Food and Drug Administration [FDA]–approved additive solution). The relatively short lifespan of a stored RBC unit results in only a few days' supply of type O blood being available at any given time in the United States. Inventory of other blood groups is generally lower, and supply of many rare types relies on dedicated procurement on an as-needed basis and a very limited inventory of frozen units.

Blood procurement is based on historical models of demand that reflect seasonal changes that are relatively consistent from year to year. Although this process is generally capable of meeting demands, it is not particularly well suited to react to unpredicted increases in demand or decreases in donor availability. Widespread natural disasters such as the 2005 hurricane Katrina have resulted in acute shortages of blood and blood products. Although these acute shortages are problematic, they are rarely so widespread or prolonged that active management of distribution cannot rectify the shortages.

A growing and somewhat inevitable problem that will impact the reliability and robustness of future blood procurement is the increasingly elderly demographic of the United States population.[1] Currently, approximately 20% of the United States population is older than 60 years. As the Baby Boom generation (those born between 1946 and 1964) reaches retirement age after 2010, the percentage of the population that is elderly will increase rapidly, and is expected to increase to 25% to 30% over the next 20 years. Increased frequencies of hematologic disorders and other degenerative disorders associated with an increasingly elderly population are expected to decrease donation rates and increase demand. These changes will not be overcome easily with distribution management.

Several recent studies[2,3] have highlighted that blood transfusion may be associated with previously unknown adverse consequences. Retrospective analyses of the ongoing health of patients that have received many transfusions of blood suggest that morbidity and mortality rates can be correlated with the storage age of the blood the patients received. Although the conclusions of these retrospective studies have been widely debated,[4] transfusing an individual with large quantities of blood containing large numbers of RBCs that have aged during storage and are approaching or exceeding their natural lifespan in vivo is intuitively detrimental. If future, large, prospective randomized trials confirm that blood cannot be stored safely for as long as currently expected, this will inevitably lead to higher demands for procurement or production of fresh blood. A shorter shelf life would also make national and international distribution increasingly challenging and provide further incentive to develop alternative and robust manufacturing methods that can be easily replicated to provide local production capabilities nationally and internationally.

Although wars are generally regarded as bloody events, improvements in body armor and battlefield tactics have made modern warfare increasingly safe for both soldiers and civilians. However, battlefield trauma is inevitable, and effective treatment necessitates a complex logistics system to maintain robust and reliable supplies of blood to the frontline. Often battles are fought in an extraterritorial manner (eg, Iraq and Afghanistan) at a considerable distance from sources of appropriately screened blood donors. Blood rarely can be procured directly within the theater of operations. Irrespective of where it is used, blood for treating United States soldiers is obtained almost exclusively from within the United States.

Because of the relatively short shelf life of blood, battlefield requirements must be predicted many days in advance to allow for procurement, screening, and subsequent distribution of blood and blood products to the battlefield or near-battlefield settings around the globe. The magnitude and impact of this logistical challenge is reflected in the interest of the Department of Defense in providing funding to develop robust and reliable methods to supply safe blood to the battlefield without the need for routine procurement in the United States (http://www.darpa.mil/dso/thrusts/bio/tactbio_med/blood_pharm/index.htm). Grant funding agencies in other countries are supporting similar initiatives for civilian use (http://www.wellcome.ac.uk/News/Media-office/Press-releases/2009/WTX054309.htm).

In recent years incremental advances in nucleic acid–based testing technologies have been useful in improving the ability to screen for established TTDs such as HIV and hepatitis B and C viruses. Improvements in these technologies, together with traditional serology, have also highlighted the increasing incidence of more novel TTDs, including arboviruses (arthropod-borne viruses), in previously unaffected populations and locations (see the article by Roger Y. Dodd elsewhere in this issue for further exploration of this topic).

In a recent public workshop,[5] the FDA evaluated the threat of arboviruses to transfusion and transplantation safety. Arboviruses such as Dengue, Japanese encephalitis, tick-borne encephalitis, Colorado tick fever, and West Nile viruses are becoming increasingly widespread. Transmission of West Nile and Dengue viruses through blood transfusion has been well documented. Dengue outbreaks have recently occurred in Texas, Hawaii, Puerto Rico, and the United States Virgin Islands. Dengue, tick-borne encephalitis, and Japanese encephalitis viruses have the potential to become endemic in certain regions of the United States. Greater understanding of the prevalence of TTD, in the absence of effective methods to eradicate causative agents, is further likely to decrease the future ability to procure safe blood and blood products.

If the increased incidence of a single TTD was a sufficient driver of change, then the rapid increase in the prevalence of HIV in the United States and around the globe in the 1980s might have been expected to provide sufficient incentive to stimulate the development of alternatives to donor procurement. Although the increased prevalence of HIV stimulated the development of novel and successful blood screening tools, it did not lead to the development of successful blood substitutes (see the article by Abdu I. Alayash elsewhere in this issue for further exploration of this topic). Arguably, the impetus for change was present, but the technology understanding to develop alternatives was not, and both were required for success.

Over the past 30 years, several innovative approaches have tried to reduce or eliminate the need for regular donation of blood for transfusion, including the development of improved storage solutions[6] or lyophilization techniques[7] to prolong the storage of whole blood, together with development of perfluorocarbon compound–based substitutes for RBC-mediated oxygenation.[8] Unfortunately despite being highly innovative, many of these approaches have failed to improve the robustness or reliability of blood supply.

Although a detailed analysis of the failure of these technologies to impact blood transfusion is outside the scope of this article, a few general observations can be made; most of the techniques that have failed have attempted to substitute natural processes with synthetic approaches. Additionally, studies in other biomedical disciplines have highlighted that while the aggregate functions of cells within tissues can be mimicked successfully with artificial substitutes, including pyrolytic carbon heart valves, Dacron vascular grafts, and Teflon components of joint prostheses, biomedical engineers have failed to successfully reverse-engineer tissues into their component parts at a cellular level. A recent explosion in regenerative medicine research is getting researchers closer to manufacturing functional tissues from sets of cellular component parts rather than merely attempting to recreate gross functions.

Recent advances in the related field of stem cell biology, combined with the cumulative impact of factors that will decrease the future availability of safe blood, are highly likely to provide the methods and the drivers for the development of transformational alternatives to transfusion with routinely donated blood.

Elsewhere in this issue, Luc Douay highlights that blood transfusion in 2020 may be based on stem cell–derived RBCs produced by tissue culture methods ex vivo. Although the development of this process is likely to be highly challenging, given the current rate of progress in stem cell biology and regenerative medicine, bioreactor design, and automation, it is reasonable to suspect that RBC manufacture may be practical by 2020. To understand how practical, and therefore how widespread this process is likely to be, it is useful to consider the current state of the art of many of the component parts that are likely to be required to make ex vivo, stem cell–based, blood product production robust and reliable.

TRANSFORMATIONAL TECHNOLOGIES: STEM CELLS, NOVEL BIOREACTORS, AND HIGH-THROUGHPUT CELL SORTING SYSTEMS
Stem Cells and the Case for CD34+ Cells

Since a spectacular debut into public awareness in 1999,[9] human embryonic stem (hES) cells have been proposed as a panacea for disorders as diverse as diabetes and facial wrinkles. More recently, advances in the preparation and culture of inducible pluripotent stem (iPS) cells[10] have further heightened the expectations surrounding the therapeutic potential of stem cells. Although recent progress in the development of many cell and stem cell–based therapies has been aided by investment and rapid advances made in hES and iPS cell technology, other stem cell populations, most importantly CD34+ stem cells, have been isolated and characterized for considerably longer.

Together with a large basic science literature, a wealth of transplant and clinical experience with CD34+ stem cells has been obtained over the past 60 years. Despite a legitimate claim to the term *stem cell* and their proven therapeutic potential, excitement about the use of CD34+ cells has recently been eclipsed by hES and iPS cells. The perceived potency that each different stem cell population exhibits likely accounts for CD34+ cells' relative lack of fame. Many embryonic stem and iPS cell lines are pluripotent (ie, they can differentiate to adopt the phenotypes of many different cell types associated with multiple germ layers). By comparison, the multipotency of

CD34+ stem cells is generally restricted to adopting differentiated characteristics of hematopoietic cells.

For many products, more is often better. For instance, consider the prominence of higher pixel counts when purchasing a digital camera, or the importance of the SUV luggage carrying capacity for the average family of four. Likewise, greater stem cell potency is often perceived to confer greater efficacy; however, when considering individual stem cell–based therapies, this is unlikely to be the case, especially when taking into account current regulatory authority positions on stem cell potency. From a regulatory perspective, the greater the potency exhibited by a stem cell population the greater the potential for uncontrolled proliferation or differentiation that may lead to malignant cell growth or ectopic tissue formation. As an example, Geron Corp., which is a pioneer in the therapeutic use of hES cell–based therapies, has been subject to protracted clinical holds while they attempt to address FDA concerns over the potential for dysregulated differentiation of their stem cell product GRNOPC1. In comparison, the safety of CD34+-derived cells has been well documented in numerous successful clinical studies. In particular, the hematopoietic lineage restriction of CD34+ cells suggests that ectopic or dysregulated tissue formation after transfusion of derived blood products would be highly unlikely.

Even though studies have shown that hES cells[11] can be transformed into hematopoietic stem cells that give rise to RBCs, the process is substantially more complex than the relatively simple expansion and RBC differentiation of a CD34+ stem cell population. With due deference to Occam's razor, addition of manipulation steps to cell-based product manufacturing protocols generally detracts from process robustness and adds cost.

Fortunately, normal human CD34+ stem cells are available from various sources. CD34+ stem cells can be isolated from bone marrow or through apheresis of peripheral blood. Apheresis is however relatively inefficient without prior bone marrow mobilization, and the invasive nature of bone marrow harvest would deter many donors if required on a routine basis. As an accessible alternative to bone marrow or peripheral blood apheresis nearly 4 million umbilical cords and placental tissues are discarded each year in the United States as a byproduct of normal full-term births. These postpartum tissues represent a readily available source of CD34+ stem cells that can be tested easily for TTD.

LifeBankUSA has pioneered perfusion approaches to extract stem cells from placental tissue in conjunction with conventional harvest of umbilical cord blood (UCB). These combined methods routinely isolate more than a billion total nucleated cells (TNC) that contain approximately 1% to 4% CD34+ stem cells. Even in the absence of additional CD34+ cells obtained from placenta perfusate, UCB represents an abundant, accessible, and noncontroversial (compared with hES cells) source of stem cells capable of expanding and differentiating in culture to RBCs.

The concept of using UCB-derived stem cells to generate RBC is not novel. Several groups have successfully achieved laboratory-scale expansion and RBC differentiation of UCB-derived stem cells.[12–14]

Large-Scale Stem Cell Culture and Novel Bioreactors

The ability to procure pluri- or multipotent stem cells in large quantities certainly enables ex vivo RBC production, but robust and reliable manufacturing processes consist of more than just effective cell isolation methods. The key challenge to manufacturing RBCs from a stem cell source is the sheer magnitude of the expansion required to generate the approximately 2×10^{12} RBCs contained in each traditional blood unit. Previous studies have highlighted that it is possible to induce

1×10^6- to 2×10^6-fold expansion of CD34+ stem cells in culture.[12,13] However, these methods relied on complex media formulations or the use of stromal cell feeder cell populations in co-culture with CD34+ stem cells. Although the use of stromal feeder layers in a clinical manufacturing process is not impossible, it would add additional complexity to reagent qualification processes for cGMP-compatible production.

Using a novel strategy of daily passaging, methods were recently developed to facilitate up to 1.5×10^6-fold expansion of peripheral blood–derived CD34+ cells in a stroma-free culture system.[15] In conjunction with enhanced CD34+ expansion methods, techniques were recently developed to ensure almost 100% differentiation efficiency of CD34+ cells to mature RBCs.[16]

A considerable gulf is often present between observations made in the laboratory and those made in the clinic. However, recent studies[17,18] indicate that previous observations of the hematopoietic potential of Notch ligand–mediated CD34+ cell expansion in vitro can safely and successfully be translated into the clinic. When considering the potential to translate the levels of expansion and differentiation of CD34+ cells in vitro in combination with the numbers of CD34+ stem cells that can be obtained from UCB and placenta perfusate, CD34+ stem cell–derived RBC manufacture seems not only possible but also increasingly practical.

Technologies that have attempted to replace RBCs with artificial substitutes have largely failed, whereas processes (eg, stem cell differentiation) that have mimicked nature have shown promise, at least on a laboratory scale. If the ability to mimic nature is extrapolated to 2020, successful RBC manufacturing processes will likely mimic the efficiency and specialized functions of bone marrow. **Fig. 1** illustrates some of the specialized functions of bone marrow and the artificial processes that could mimic these functions. Although experts can reasonably predict that future RBC manufacture will use stem cells (most likely CD34+ cells) as a raw material, what expansion and differentiation methodologies will be used is less clear. Through referencing the current knowledge and comparisons with the functions and composition of bone marrow, one can predict that stem cell differentiation likely will be based on the combined actions of mitogens and cytokines such as interleukin-3, erythropoietin, and stem cell factor.[13] If moderate differentiation efficiency ($\sim$50%) is assumed, then each unit of RBCs will require the production of 4×10^{12} cells before differentiation. Furthermore, before harvest, approximately 4×10^{12} cells must be sorted to obtain a relatively pure population of terminally differentiated cells highly enriched for RBC.

When deciding between hES or iPS cells versus CD34+ cells as raw materials for RBC manufacture, the effects of cell density on the required culture systems is important to consider. hES and iPS cells are normally adherent and require attachment to a substratum to proliferate. Current embryonic stem cell culture conditions dictate that these cells be maintained at a maximal density of 1×10^6 cells/cm^2 or less. At these densities, approximately 400 m^2 (approximately the size of 2 tennis courts) of growth area would be required to culture 4×10^{12} cells before differentiation. Approximately 160 large-format (40 tray) cell factories and approximately 1200 L of growth medium would be required to achieve and support this surface area; a situation that is clearly untenable.

Using microcarriers to support the growth of these adherent cells would significantly improve the situation. Theoretically, approximately 166 L of medium containing approximately 6.6 g of Cytodex microcarriers (Sigma-Aldrich Co, St Louis, MI, USA) could provide a surface area of 400 m^2. Although this is an improvement over cell factories, it still represents a significant, and most likely unbearable, cost burden per unit of RBCs. Cell factories, and to a lesser extent microcarriers, are still woefully

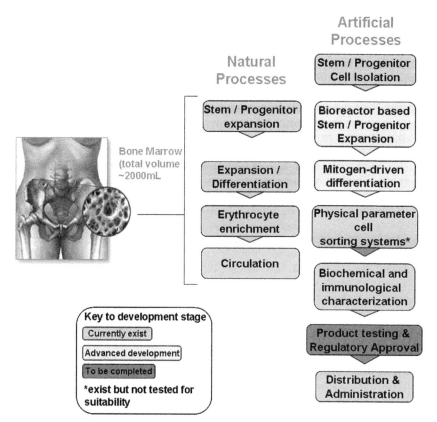

Fig. 1. Key functions of adult bone marrow in red blood cell (RBC) manufacture contrasted with an overview the substitute process steps that would be required to manufacture RBC ex vivo. Some of the substitute processes currently exist, and others are in advanced development, having been proven in medium- to large-scale laboratory settings. Still others will need to be initiated and completed before the practical implementation of an ex vivo manufactured RBC in a clinical setting.

inefficient compared with the manufacturing capacity of bone marrow. A volume approximating 2 L of adult human bone marrow can generate up to 9×10^9 cells per hour.

The large space and reagent requirements necessary for the growth of hES or iPS cells seem to prohibit efficient RBC production, but can nonadherent CD34+ cells be any more effective? Given that they have no dependency on substratum attachment for proliferation, the maximum growth density of nonadherent cells in culture largely depends on the efficiency of the culture system in supporting diffusion-limited exchange of nutrients, waste products, and gases across all parts of the system. Conventional "stirred tank" or agitated bag-based bioreactors represent the state of the art of commonly used nonadherent culture systems. These systems can generally support cell densities of approximately 1×10^7 cells/mL; however at these densities a minimum of 400 L of medium would be required to support nonadherent CD34+ cell growth.

Laboratory-scale, two-compartment hollow fiber-based bioreactors, such as those supplied by FiberCell Systems, can support nonadherent cell densities of approximately 1×10^8 cells/mL (Frederick, MD, USA; http://www.fibercellsystems. com). These bioreactors are comprised of a cell compartment, situated between the hollow fibers, and a combined unidirectional gas and medium compartment within the lumen of the hollow fibers.

Although these systems are substantially less efficient than bone marrow, they are approaching the realm of feasibility in requiring approximately 40 L of medium to support the maximum predifferentiation cell densities for each unit of RBCs produced. Further development and optimization of two-compartment hollow fiber bioreactors might be expected to increase their efficiency; however, because of an inherent design limitation, two-compartment hollow fibers may be incapable of being developed to a point where they can support cost-effective ex vivo RBC production (ie, support of cell growth densities approaching 1×10^9 cells/mL).

Nutrient and waste-product exchange in two-compartment devices, such as the FiberCell Systems Duet pump (FiberCell Systems, Frederick, MD, USA), in which cells are distributed around a bundle of hollow fibers, is limited by nonuniform mass exchange with large substrate gradients. Oxygen supply together with carbon dioxide exchange, and thus pH regulation through bicarbonate-based buffer systems, must be provided by external gas exchangers/oxygenators, which add complexity and lead to large gradients within the bioreactors. This nonuniformity not only limits the cell growth density but can also lead to heterogeneous stem cell expansion and subsequent differentiation.

In vivo, stem cells are exquisitely sensitive to substrate and morphogenic cues that drive their proliferation or lineage commitment. In vitro, most stem cell populations are uniquely susceptible to subtle changes in their culture environments. These changes can substantially alter their proliferative or differentiated phenotypes. To maintain uniform growth conditions and achieve higher cell growth densities, medium and gas exchange within the conventional hollow fiber bioreactors must be improved. To provide a more uniform mass exchange with low gradients, two-compartment hollow fiber systems must be replaced by three-compartment systems. If internal gas exchange with low gradients is required, a fourth compartment is necessary.[19]

Several recent advances were made in the design of liver cell bioreactors for extracorporeal organ assist devices that may positively impact future approaches to RBC manufacture.[20] In particular, an acute shortage of donor tissues for transplantation combined with a lack of conventional therapeutic approaches for liver failure has driven the development of several innovative approaches to bioengineered liver support devices.

For example, the clinically relevant four-compartment bioreactor developed by Jörg Gerlach,[21] now produced by Stem Cell Systems (SCS; Berlin, Germany; http://www. stemcell-systems.com) as a potential ex vivo liver assist device, may well represent a practical solution to growing stem cells at densities compatible with cost-effective RBC manufacture. Each of the SCS bioreactors (**Fig. 2**) contains two bundles of hollow fibers for transport of culture medium (forming two medium compartments), interwoven with one bundle of oxygenation membranes for transport of oxygen and carbon dioxide (the gas compartment), with cells being cultured in the spaces between the fibers (the fourth cell compartment). Interweaving the fibers into a regular pattern of identical subunits allows decentralized mass exchange and reduction of gradients. The composition of the fibers allows most proteins to pass freely through the fiber walls and into the cell compartment. Using countercurrent flow, medium can be pumped through the medium compartments in opposing directions, ensuring that the medium in the cell compartment is well mixed. The ability to maintain a homogeneous environment in all parts of the bioreactor is critical for process optimization and robustness and for uniform control of stem cell proliferation and differentiation.

A
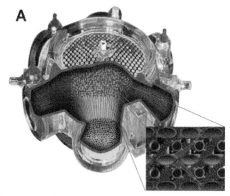

B
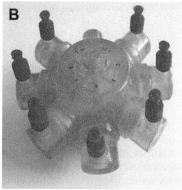

Fig. 2. (A) Schematic of the bioreactor housing and independent fiber bundles, interwoven to form a multicompartment space for cell culture, highlighting the potential for independent cell, gas, and counter-current medium exchange. (B) Photograph of an assembled small-scale four-compartment bioreactor system (perfusion apparatus not shown).

This type of four-compartment bioreactor system is currently and reliably capable of supporting CD34+ cell densities up to 1×10^8 cells/mL (J. Gerlach, personal communication, 2009). However, given the inherent design advantages over two-compartment systems, experts believe that further modification of medium and gas compositions cell densities could enhance this density a further fourfold. Cell growth densities approaching 1×10^9 are comparable to bone marrow and may facilitate robust and cost-effective ex vivo stem cell production for RBC manufacture.

Differentiation Efficiency and Red Blood Cell Enrichment Strategies

Reliable and efficient stem cell isolation and expansion represent two of the three critical steps during ex vivo RBC manufacture. The final step (before safety and efficacy assessment and regulatory approval) is to ensure that the expanded populations can be differentiated with near 100% efficiently. Alternatively, if the frequency of RBC differentiation is significantly less than 100%, robust mechanisms must exist to purify RBCs from the resulting mixed cell population.

Douay and Giarratana[16] recently reported techniques to drive stem cell–derived RBC differentiation to near 100% in laboratory-scale studies. However, the efficiency of this process relies on a multistep expansion/differentiation protocol using growth factor–rich medium and stromal feeder cells followed by removal of major growth factors. More simple approaches often trade simplicity for differentiation efficiency. Stromal cell–independent methods, as exemplified by the work of Boehm and colleagues,[15] often lead to less-effective terminal differentiation (ie, ~40%–50% enucleation).

From a manufacturing perspective, trading off RBC differentiation efficiency for simple cost-effective and more easily cGMP-compatible expansion/differentiation processes may be preferable, especially if stem cell isolation (feedstock) and expansion protocols are highly effective and can be coupled with effective RBC enrichment strategies as a product polishing step.

Many methods currently exist to enrich or purify RBCs from a mixed population. Conventional fluorescence-activated cell sorting (FACS) can be used to discriminate and sort RBCs based on size or fluorescently tagged surface marker expression profiles. Unfortunately, although these methods can be extremely effective, they are relatively slow. Current high-speed FACS systems can be operated at rates of approximately 5×10^4 sorting events per second, therefore 4×10^{12} cells containing 50% RBCs would require approximately 900 days to sort. The unique size and specific density distributions together with the highly deformable nature of mature RBCs could also be exploited to enrich mixed populations.

Many clinical systems currently exist to enrich RBCs, some as a desired characteristic of the process, and others as a byproduct of extracting stem cell populations or leukodepletion. Size, surface area, and charge-based filtration are often used to leukodeplete cellular blood products in the blood bank. Although filtration can result in small amounts of hemolysis, these systems can rapidly process large numbers of cells and could be adapted for RBC purification. Likewise, batch-mode centrifugation and continuous centrifugal elutriation methods are currently used to debulk RBCs from cord blood during clinical stem cell harvesting procedures or processing (eg, AXP AutoXpress system; ThermoGenesis Corp, Rancho Cordova, CA, USA) and devices such as the Baxter-Fenwal CS-3000 system (Fenwal Inc, Lake Zurich, IL, USA) can extract various blood products during clinical apheresis procedures. These systems may be adaptable for use in RBC manufacturing processes.

In addition to the specific density and size differences of RBCs compared with stem cell populations, another unique property of mature RBC may also be exploited. Because of their high iron-containing hemoglobin content, RBCs, especially when deoxygenated, exhibit a distinct magnetic susceptibility compared with other cell types or water.[22] The practical use of these observations was shown through the capture of erythrocytes, deoxygenated with a sodium dithionite solution, on a ferromagnetic wire mesh that produced a high gradient magnetic field induced by an external field.[23]

More recently, Zborowski and colleagues[24] further defined how the magnetophoretic properties of RBCs can be exploited for characterization and sorting. Advanced microfluidic devices have been used to show high-efficiency sorting of RBCs.[25,26] The current throughput of these devices is relatively low (5–13 μL/h) and would be incompatible with large-scale RBC productions if not for the possibility of using printed circuit–type microfabrication techniques to produce a massively parallel microfluidic-based system capable of processing much larger volumes.

Given the availability of current and rapidly developing technologies suitable for large-scale RBC purification, this process will probably not pose significant challenges to the future development of ex vivo RBC manufacturing systems. Additionally, if used in conjunction with heterogeneous nonadherent stem and RBC cell populations, many of the techniques outlined earlier could facilitate recovery of uncommitted stem cells capable of being further maintained in the bioreactor system as part of a more continuous process.

Regulatory Considerations

As outlined in **Fig. 1** and elsewhere in this article, when considering mimicking bone marrow function ex vivo in a robust and reliable manner, regulatory challenges must be considered in addition to the scientific hurdles. The benefits of process and reagent simplicity in aiding cGMP-compatibility have already been highlighted, but to determine whether achieving routine clinical implementation of an ex vivo–manufactured RBC will be possible within the next decade, the likely route to product approval must be considered from a regulatory perspective. Although CD34+ stem cells are currently used as a key component of hematopoietic stem cell transplantation procedures, hES cell-based therapies are still awaiting formal clinical safety and efficacy trials. Clinical trials of a new therapeutic agent can take at least 5 years to complete.

Table 1
Selected factors that may accelerate or delay regulatory approval of ex vivo–manufactured red blood cells

Accelerate	Delay
CD34+ stem cell–based therapies have a long and relatively safe clinical history	hES and iPS cell–derived therapies represent new classes of therapeutic agents that will require extensive preclinical and clinical safety testing to be deemed safe
The terminally differentiated and enucleated phenotype of mature RBC suggests that tumorogenic change of a purified population is highly unlikely	Stem cell–based therapies that include novel manufacturing devices are likely to require approvals for both the product and the manufacturing devices
Unlike many other potential stem cell-based products, a well characterized gold standard (venopuncture-derived RBCs) exists that could facilitate the comparison of ex vivo–manufactured RBC characteristics	The characteristics of stem cell-derived RBC may not be identical to venopuncture-derived RBCs; therefore, the degree comparability may require extensive interpretation
Many well-validated and accepted tests of RBC function exist	Currently, stem cell-derived blood products could fall under the two offices within the FDA: Office for Cell and Gene Therapy and the Office for Blood and Blood Products
Support from federal agencies, such as the United States Department of Defense and the UK Blood Transfusion Service, may provide pump-priming funds for early development	The relatively low value (reimbursement) associated with donor-derived RBCs may challenge the development of a commercially viable business case to support manufacture

Even when the therapeutic class of the new therapeutic agent under study is well understood, clinical trials can be protracted. Therefore, clinical trials of hES cell–based therapies probably will be further extended because of the relative lack of knowledge of the cellular feedstock.

Many factors may accelerate or delay the approval of an ex vivo–manufactured RBC product; certain key considerations are listed in **Table 1**. On balance, if an ex vivo–manufactured RBC product is to gain regulatory approval in the United States before 2020, it will need to be developed sufficiently to allow clinical trials to start within the next few years. As highlighted previously, given the current Department of Defense (Defense Advanced Research Projects Agency) wish to be able to show practical solutions for RBC manufacture in the near future, these timelines look increasingly realistic.

SUMMARY

Transformative changes in blood transfusion practices have been relatively rare in the past century. Recently several factors, including increasing elderly demographics, and increasing prevalence of TTD, recently have combined to provide drivers for further innovation in the field. Advances in stem cell biology and bioreactor design are likely to underpin the development of transformational alternatives to traditional approaches to blood transfusion. Considering the state of development of CD34+ cell–based therapeutics and the rates of change in clinically compatible hardware systems, it is reasonable to believe that stem cell–based ex vivo production of RBC will be routine, robust, and reliable within the next decade.

ACKNOWLEDGMENTS

Bioreactor images and information were provided courtesy of Drs Jörg Gerlach and Greggory Housler, at the University of Pittsburgh.

REFERENCES

1. Campbell PR. Population projections of the United States by age, sex, race and Hispanic origin: 1995 to 2050. Washington, DC: U.S. Bureau of the Census, Current Population Reports; 1996. p. 25.
2. Spinella PC, Carroll CL, Staff I, et al. Duration of red blood cell storage is associated with increased incidence of deep vein thrombosis and in hospital mortality in patients with traumatic injuries. Crit Care 2009;13(5):R151.
3. Koch CG, Li L, Sessler DI, et al. Duration of red-cell storage and complications after cardiac surgery. N Engl J Med 2008;358(12):1229–39.
4. Triulzi DJ, Yazer MH. Clinical studies of the effect of blood storage on patient outcomes. Transfus Apher Sci, in press.
5. U.S. Food and Drug Administration. Public Workshop. Emerging arboviruses: evaluating the threat to transfusion and transplantation safety. Bethesda (MD), December 14–15, 2009.
6. Davey RJ, Carmen RA, Simon TL, et al. Preparation of white cell-depleted red cells for 42-day storage using an integral in-line filter. Transfusion 1989;29(6):496–9.
7. Han Y, Quan GB, Liu XZ, et al. Improved preservation of human red blood cells by lyophilization. Cryobiology 2005;51(2):152–64.
8. Cole RP, Wittenberg BA, Caldwell PR. Myoglobin function in the isolated fluorocarbon-perfused dog heart. Am J Physiol 1978;234(5):H567–72.
9. Stem cells named breakthrough of the year. Science 1999.
10. Takahashi K, Yamanaka S. Induction of pluripotent stem cells from mouse embryonic and adult fibroblast cultures by defined factors. Cell 2006;126(4):663–76.
11. Vodyanik MA, Bork JA, Thomson JA, et al. Human embryonic stem cell-derived CD34+ cells: efficient production in the coculture with OP9 stromal cells and analysis of lymphohematopoietic potential. Blood 2005;105(2):617–26.
12. Neildez-Nguyen TM, Wajcman H, Marden MC, et al. Human erythroid cells produced *ex vivo* at large scale differentiate into red blood cells *in vivo*. Nat Biotechnol 2002;20(5):467–72.
13. Giarratana MC, Kobari L, Lapillonne H, et al. *Ex vivo* generation of fully mature human red blood cells from hematopoietic stem cells. Nat Biotechnol 2005; 23(1):69–74.
14. Baek EJ, Kim HS, Kim S, et al. In vitro clinical-grade generation of red blood cells from human umbilical cord blood CD34+ cells. Transfusion 2008;48(10): 2235–45.
15. Boehm D, Murphy WG, Al-Rubeai M. The potential of human peripheral blood derived CD34+ cells for *ex vivo* red blood cell production. J Biotechnol 2009; 144(2):127–34.
16. Douay L, Giarratana MC. *Ex vivo* generation of human red blood cells: a new advance in stem cell engineering. Methods Mol Biol 2009;482:127–40.
17. Delaney C, Varnum-Finney B, Aoyama K, et al. Dose-dependent effects of the Notch ligand Delta1 on ex vivo differentiation and in vivo marrow repopulating ability of cord blood cells. Blood 2005;106(8):2693–9.
18. Delaney C, Heimfeld S, Brashem-Stein C, et al. Notch-mediated expansion of human cord blood progenitor cells capable of rapid myeloid reconstitution. Nat Med 2010;16(2):232–6.

19. Gerlach JC, Zeilinger K, Patzer Ii JF. Bioartificial liver systems: why, what, whither? Regen Med 2008;3(4):575–95.
20. Monga SP, Hout MS, Baun MJ, et al. Mouse fetal liver cells in artificial capillary beds in three-dimensional four-compartment bioreactors. Am J Pathol 2005; 167(5):1279–92.
21. Sauer IM, Kardassis D, Zeillinger K, et al. Clinical extracorporeal hybrid liver support–phase I study with primary porcine liver cells. Xenotransplantation 2003;10(5):460–9.
22. Pauling L, Coryell CD. The magnetic properties and structure of hemoglobin, oxyhemoglobin and carbonmonoxyhemoglobin. Proc Natl Acad Sci U S A 1936;22(4):210–6.
23. Melville D. Direct magnetic separation of red cells from whole blood. Nature 1975; 255(5511):706.
24. Zborowski M, Ostera GR, Moore LR, et al. Red blood cell magnetophoresis. Biophys J 2003;84(4):2638–45.
25. Han KH, Frazier AB. Paramagnetic capture mode magnetophoretic microseparator for high efficiency blood cell separations. Lab Chip 2006;6(2):265–73.
26. Qu BY, Wu ZY, Fang F, et al. A glass microfluidic chip for continuous blood cell sorting by a magnetic gradient without labeling. Anal Bioanal Chem 2008; 392(7–8):1317–24.

Future of Molecular Testing for Red Blood Cell Antigens

Joann M. Moulds, PhD, MT(ASCP)SBB

KEYWORDS

• Red cell antigens • Genotyping • Microarray

When one looks at the field of molecular pathology or transplantation, it is evident that molecular biology has made a positive impact on medicine. However, the progress in transfusion medicine has been slower and more cautious than in other areas of the clinical laboratory. The US Food and Drug Administration (FDA)-sponsored "Workshop on Molecular Methods in Immunohematology"[1] and the publication of the first edition of the AABB Standards for Molecular Testing for Red Cell, Platelet, and Neutrophil Antigens[2] give witness that change has begun and change will continue. To understand where the field may go in the next 10 years requires that the reader understand what technology is available now. Therefore, this article discusses the current state of the art for red cell genotyping and newer, ever-evolving molecular technologies. Because it is impossible to present all of the molecular techniques and their variations in this article, the author selects a group of methodologies to review and speculates where the field of molecular immunohematology may be in 2020.

DETECTION OF RED CELL BLOOD GROUP POLYMORPHISMS

Blood group antigens are inherited polymorphisms found on the red blood cell, but may also occur on other cells and in secretions. Since the discovery of the ABH blood group at the beginning of the twentieth century, more than 300 red cell antigens have been identified and placed into 30 distinct blood-group systems.[3] Until recently, blood group antigens were only detected by hemagglutination methods. However, following the advent of molecular technology, the majority of the blood group genes were identified, sequenced, and single nucleotide polymorphisms (SNPs) assigned to blood group antigen specificities. These molecular findings were followed closely by the development of laboratory defined tests (LDT) and later commercial assays for the prediction of red cell phenotypes by DNA methods. Presently, there are no US FDA-approved molecular technologies for red cell blood group genotyping and most commercial kits are being sold for Research Use Only. Some of these molecular

Clinical Immunogenetics, LifeShare Blood Centers, 8910 Linwood Avenue, Shreveport, LA 71106, USA
E-mail address: jmmoulds@lifeshare.org

Clin Lab Med 30 (2010) 419–429
doi:10.1016/j.cll.2010.02.004
0272-2712/10/$ – see front matter © 2010 Elsevier Inc. All rights reserved.

labmed.theclinics.com

test methods are presented, but the reader should be aware that the field of molecular immunohematology is rapidly changing as better molecular methods are developed making it impossible to cover every permutation in this article.

Available Test Methods

The molecular methods currently available for red cell genotyping can be divided into two categories: (1) low to medium-throughput and (2) high-throughput. The former can be useful in a hospital or reference-lab setting where patient samples (including fetal DNA) are being individually tested, whereas high-throughput testing is best done in a donor center where large-volume screening can be performed. Many of the low-throughput methods employ polymerase chain reaction (PCR) and these can be set up easily in the lab. Several adaptations of the basic PCR technology have been made and they are described later.

Low-throughput methods

The earliest LDTs used PCR to amplify specific regions of the target blood group gene. The PCR product or amplicon could then be cut with a known restriction enzyme and the DNA fragments visualized on an agarose gel. The band pattern was dependent on whether a restriction site was lost or gained when the blood group SNP was present. For example, the Tc^b antigen results from a base pair change of 155G>C resulting in the gain of a restriction site. As seen in **Fig. 1**, amplicon from a Tc(a+b+) person demonstrates an uncut band of 300 bp (Tc^a) using *Stu*I but two new bands appear if Tc^b is present. Obviously, these types of assays can be very subjective.

Another, somewhat faster adaptation of the basic PCR method is PCR-SSP (sequence-specific primer) or allele-specific PCR (AS-PCR), which omits the restriction digest step. In this assay, a primer that only detects the allele of interest is used in the PCR and a band is observed on the gel only when the gene of interest is present (**Fig. 2**). Wagner and colleagues[4] reported the use of a multiplex PCR-SSP that they used to screen for donors who were negative for the following high-incidence antigens: Kp^b, Co^a, Yt^a and Lu^b. In addition to LDTs, there are commercially available kits that can be used to test for *RHD* variants and other blood group genes such as *K1/K2, FYA/FYB,* and *JKA/JKB*. In general, these methods are labor intensive and can only test a few samples at a time, thus, they are not suitable for large-scale genotyping but lend themselves well to a reference lab or hospital setting.

Medium-throughput methods

Other methods that are considered as medium-throughput use real-time PCR. This procedure follows the general principle of PCR but its key feature is that the amplified DNA is detected as the reaction progresses in *real time*. In general, there are two common methods for detection of products using real-time PCR: (1) non-specific

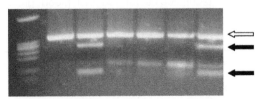

Fig. 1. A PCR-RFLP using the restriction enzyme *Stu*I to detect the Cromer blood group alleles *TCA* and *TCB*. The open arrow indicates a Tc^a-specific band, and the dark errors indicate the restriction fragments associated with the Tc^b phenotype.

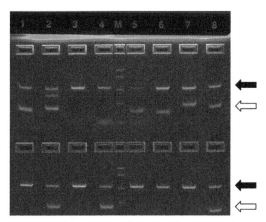

Fig. 2. A commercially available AS-PCR for the detection of *RHD* (GTI Diagnostics, Waukesha, Wisconsin). Internal positive control (*dark arrows*) and Allele-specific reactions (*open arrows*). M, marker.

fluorescent dyes that intercalate with any double-stranded DNA (SYBR Green [Applied Biosystems, Foster City, CA, USA]); and (2) sequence-specific DNA probes consisting of oligonucleotides that are labeled with a fluorescent reporter that permits detection only after hybridization of the probe with its complementary DNA target (TaqMan [Applied Biosystems, Foster City, CA, USA]). The first has been used in combination with various instruments (eg, Lightcycler [Roche, Indianapolis, IN, USA] and ABI 7500 [Applied Biosystems, Foster City, CA, USA] to detect *RH 1-5* [D, C/c, E/e]; *JK1/2*; and *KEL1/2*).[5]

Some other medium throughput assays are real-time PCR with melting-curve analysis and pyrosequencing. Until recently melting and analysis of the entire PCR product was not generally successful at finding single-base variants. However, with higher-resolution instruments and advanced dyes, amplicon melting analysis of a single SNP is now possible with several instruments. Detection of red cell blood group SNPs by melting-curve analysis has been used to genotype for *KEL1/2, JK1/2, FY1/2, FY0, FYX, MNS1-4, DO1/2, CO1/2, LU1/2, YTA/B*, and *DIA/DIB*.[6–9]

Pyrosequencing is a method of DNA sequencing based on the sequencing-by-synthesis principle. It differs from the common Sanger sequencing relying on the detection of pyrophosphate release on nucleotide incorporation, rather than chain termination with dideoxynucleotides. Pyrosequencing has been successfully used for some red cell genotyping but presently is limited to a only few blood group systems including Kell, Duffy, and Kidd.[10]

High-throughput methods

The Human Genome Project forced the improvement of methods and technology for the detection of SNPs consequently reducing the cost. This improvement, paired with the identification of the red cell blood groups, has made the idea of high-throughput genotyping a reality. Several commercially available microarray-based genotyping systems being used include BLOODchip (Progenika, Derio,Vizcaya, Spain); HEA BeadChip (BioArraySolutions/Immucor, Warren, NJ, USA); and SNPstream (Beckman Coulter, Brea, CA, USA).

BLOODchip was developed by a consortium of European labs[1] and is based on a multiplex PCR method as described by Beiboer[11] The BLOODchip is a glass slide onto which probes have been spotted. A multiplex PCR is performed, the products are added to the slide, and a fluorescent dye is incorporated during the allele-specific hybridization process. It can be used to the following blood group genes: *ABH*; *MNS*; *RHD*; *RHCE*; *KE*; *FY* (including the silencing mutation); *JK*; *DI*; *DO*;*CO*.

Two microarrays that use a multiplex PCR followed by oligonucleotide elongation/extension are the HEA and the SNPstream systems, respectively. HEA uses colorized beads affixed to a chip on a slide to which the appropriate probes have been attached (**Fig. 3**). A multiplex PCR is performed, and following several intermediate steps, the product is added to the bead chip and elongation occurs with incorporation of a fluorescent tag.[12] HEA does not type for *ABH* or *RHD* (a separate chip will be available to type for D, weak D, and D variants) but does include the following genes: *RHC*; *K1/K*; *KPA/KPB*; *JSA/JSB*; *FYA/FYB* (including silencing mutation and FYX); *JKA/JKB*; *MNS* (including S silencing mutations); *LUA/LUB*; *DIA/DIB*; *COA/COB*; *DOA/DOB*; *HY*; *JOA*; *LWA/LWB*; *SC1/SC2*; and hemoglobin S. The assay can be run on an eight-chip or on a 96-chip slide plate in 5 to 6 hours, which makes the later adaptable to automation.[13]

Some of the high-throughput assays have been used mainly outside of the United States. In Canada, the Genome Lab SNPstream is being used by HemaQuebec to genotype an initial cohort of 20,000 repeat blood donors.[14] The method is based on a multiplex PCR followed by a single-base extension reaction using a gene-specific, tag-specific primer. A fluorescent label is incorporated and hybridization occurs in 384 well plates; however, the assay time is 36 hours. The initial report of more than 10,000 donors showed more than 99% concordancy with serology.[14–16]

Evolving Molecular Technologies

The assays discussed earlier are presently being produced commercially and used in labs throughout the United States, Canada, or Europe. Other molecular techniques that are under development and may be available for red cell genotyping in the next decade include fluidic or open microarrays; matrix-assisted laser desorption/ionization time-of-flight mass spectrometry (MALDI-TOF MS); and mini-sequencing or SNaPshot (Applied Biosystems, Foster City, CA, USA).

Fluidic microarray systems that could easily be available in the near future for red cell genotyping are Luminex xMAP (Luminex Corporation, Austin, TX, USA) and Open-Array (BioTrove, Woburn, MA, USA). These systems have been in use for other genotyping protocols (eg, Luminex xMap to type HLA genes) but they are just now being looked at for red cell genotyping (Gen-Probe). Luminex is a microsphere-based technology that detects PCR-amplified targets by direct hybridization to microspheres

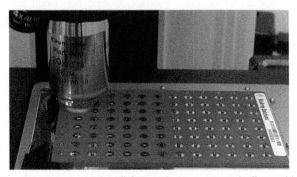

Fig. 3. Bead-chip microarray in a 96-well format being automatically read by a fluorescent microscope. (*Courtesy of* BioArray Solutions, Ltd, Warren, NJ; with permission.)

coupled to allele-specific oligonucleotides. It can analyze up to 100 different analytes in a single reaction using a flow cytometer. Karpasitou and colleagues[17] adapted the technology to type for *JKA/JKB, FYA/FYB, S/s, K1/K2, KPA/KPB/JSA/JSB, COA/ COB*, and *LUA/LUB*. Its flexibility and adaptability will be an asset for future development.

The other fluidic system that has been available but not previously used for red cell genotyping is the OpenArray by BioTrove. Initially the assay was adapted by Hopp and colleagues[18] to screen predominantly African American (A-A) blood donors for the following antigens: E/e, Fy^a/Fy^b, Jk^a/Jk^b, Lu^a/Lu^b, K/k, Js^a/Js^b, Do^a/Do^b, Jo^a, and Hy. Additional studies, including triplicate testing of 427 A-A donors, have shown more than 99% concordance with serology.[19] One advantage of the OpenArray platform is the user-specified target selection so that the platform can be adapted to screen specific ethnic groups.

Another method that may be applicable to red cell genotyping uses mass spectrometry. MALDI-TOF MS consists of two parts: (1) laser-induced desorption/ionization of analyte/matrix molecules and (2) separation and analysis of different biomolecules based on intrinsic physical properties. It is a high-throughput, qualitative, and quantitative method that can analyze 36 to 40 multiple SNPS in a single reaction that takes approximately 8 hours. It has been reported for the genotyping of some of the Kell system genes and platelet antigens.[20] Using the Sequenom platform, a prenatal screening test for fetal *RHD* has been reported with claims of more than 99% sensitivity.[21] However, the current high instrument cots may limit its availability and use in the future.

Finally, a platform that shows promise for future development in red cell genotyping is mini-sequencing or the SNaPshot assay (Applied Biosystems, Foster City, CA, USA). Cyclic mini-sequencing reactions with fluorescently labeled dideoxynucleotides are performed in solution using multiplex PCR product as template and detection primers that are designed to anneal immediately adjacent and upstream of the SNP site. Following the hybridization and extension steps, the fluorescent signals from the array are measured and the genotypes are deduced by cluster analysis. Because this assay can be performed in a 96 well plate, it could also be adapted for automation.

A mini-sequencing method to genotype the ABH blood group system has been described and found to be a reproducible strategy to type for the most common ABH alleles.[22] It is more rapid than PCR-restriction fragment length polymorphism (RFLP) and newly discovered mutations could be readily investigated by the addition of new extension primers into the mini-sequencing multiplex reaction. More recently, the SNapShot method has been used for typing for the following antigens: Fy^a/Fy^b, Do^a/Do^b, Jo^a, Hy, LW^a/LW^b, Co^a/Co^b, Sc1/Sc2, Di^a/Di^b, Jk^a/Jk^b, Lu^a/Lu^b, MNSs, and K/k.[23] This assay used three multiplex amplifications to determine 17 SNPs resulting in a throughput of 32 samples in 12 hours.

GENOTYPING COSTS

The success of any new technology is that the cost becomes reasonable compared with the benefits. For laboratories that already have basic molecular equipment, such as thermal cyclers, investment costs may be minimal. But equipment costs must be a major consideration for those newly embarking into the field, especially if automated methods become available. High cost has been cited as a reason for not doing genotyping but this argument has been recently challenged.[24,25] With the rising costs of serologic reagents and a decreasing trained work force, the introduction of automated genotyping platforms may arrive at the right time for their general acceptance.

It is difficult to make current cost comparisons between serologic and molecular methods. Some of the DNA-based methods described earlier can cost as little as $2 per SNP.[4,23] There are now reports in the literature showing that genotyping (excluding equipment costs) can be less expensive than serology with a large amount of savings being technologist time.[26,27] Of course similar savings will be dependent on local salaries and any institutional purchasing agreements. If assays are developed that target specific ethnic groups or allow the user to choose the genes that are most relevant to their patient population, then molecular typing may become very attractive to large hospitals and blood centers.

APPLICATIONS OF RED CELL GENOTYPING
Patient Genotyping

Although the ideal transfusion in the future may include matching of all patients to donors for the most clinically relevant systems (ie, ABH, RH, KEL, FY, JK, MNS), today's reality is that this is not entirely possible (**Box 1**). Thus, the focus for providing genotype-matched donors has been limited to certain patient groups including (1) chronically transfused patients (eg, aplastic anemia, sickle cell disease [SCD]); (2) patients who have produced multiple alloantibodies (especially recently transfused patients); and (3) patients having warm autoimmune hemolytic anemia (WAIHA).

The argument for and against phenotype matching of blood donors and patients has been ongoing for the last 20 years. Arguments against matching cite cost as a major drawback.[25,28] However, the Stroke Prevention Trials in Sickle Cell Anemia clinical trials have provided convincing evidence that prophylactic transfusion of C/c, E/e, and K1 matched blood helps prevent stroke and alloimmunization in patients with SCD.[29] The National Institutes of Health now recommend phenotype matching for multiply transfused patients with SCD (http://www.nhlbi.nih.gov/health/prof/blood/sickle/sc_mngt.pdf). Because of limited resources, many labs are beginning to adopt a two-tiered approach to genotype matching. All patients who are chronically transfused are matched for C, E, and K1 (limited phenotype), which is usually not difficult to achieve. However, some provide more fully (extended) matched units, once patients produce an alloantibody. At that point, large-scale genotyping of donors becomes a necessity to economically provide matched blood. Thus, we will see

---

Box 1
Applications for molecular testing of red cell antigens

1. Typing of patients and donors for antigens to which there are no available antisera

2. Typing of patients and donors for antigens when the available antibodies are weak or are in limited supply

3. Detection of genes that result in weakened antigens

4. Resolution of serologic typing discrepancies

5. Identification of an antigen positive fetus who may be at risk for hemolytic disease

6. Determining a phenotype for patients with strongly positive direct antiglobulin tests

7. Determining a phenotype for patients who have been recently transfused

8. Large scale screening of donors to provide genotyped matched units or to find donors with red cells that lack high incidence antigens

continued growth in this area until which time a sufficient number of donors have been genotyped and then donor genotyping will most likely plateau.[14]

For patients who are recently transfused and producing all antibodies, red cell genotyping is an invaluable tool. Serologic methods are tedious and may not be effective in determining patients' correct phenotype. Because many of the existing platforms can genotype for antigens for which there is a limited source (ie, anti-Do^a/Do^b), genotyping can assist in the correct identification of antibody specificities. Genotype-matched units can then be selected to be negative for patients' antibodies or more ideally to be a complete match with the major systems.

Genotyping is changing the way immunohematologists approach the identification and treatment of patients with WAIHA. Published data suggest that 25% to 40% of patients diagnosed with WAIHA may have alloantibodies that are masked by strong autoantibodies.[30] Multiple serologic techniques requiring advanced skills are often needed to investigate these cases and transfusion can be risky. Again, a genotype provides the best type, and units of blood can be selected to be a genotype match. Although the units may still be crossmatch incompatible, genotype-matched units are probably the safest blood to transfuse.

There is little argument that the provision of genotyped-matched units is advantageous for the patients just described. However, there remains skepticism for the application of genotyped-matched donors for all transfusions.[24] Perhaps a reasonable second step would be the use of genotyped-matched units for women of child-bearing age so as to decrease the risk for hemolytic disease of the fetus and newborn in the future.

Strategies for Donor Screening

The reasons for mass donor screening are simple: (1) to find blood donors having rare phenotypes, and (2) to find donors who have a combination of blood-group factors often needed for patients having multiple alloantibodies. The definition of a rare donor may vary from country to country but in general it is less than 1:1000.[31] Therefore, future molecular assays must be adaptable to screen blood donors of different ethnic backgrounds. For example, an assay that could easily screen for *JK* (null) alleles, found more frequently in the Pacific rim, would be advantageous for screening Asians but of less interest for screening Caucasians. Thus, platforms that are more flexible and user friendly may become more prominent in the blood bank market.

Actual screening strategies may also vary between blood centers. Some are only screening select ethnic groups (ie, African Americans, to supply matched units for alloimmunized patients with SCD). Others may only screen blood group O or donors that have donated three or more times. Still other centers are serologically screening for selected RH phenotypes (eg, R$_1$R$_1$) and then genotyping those donors. It is unlikely that all donors of all ABO types will ever be genotyped because it would not be cost effective.

FUTURE TRENDS AND CHALLENGES

At this point the authors have been discussing the evolution and current use of molecular methods in transfusion medicine. But what can we expect in 10 years from now? Will serology be dead? Will DNA reign supreme? Let us take a provocative look into the crystal ball.

Serologist have often been told that a genotype is not a phenotype and that there are cases where a gene may be present but not expressed on the red cell. Two common examples are the GATA-promoter polymorphism, which silences the *FYB* gene, and two different *GYPB* mutations that silence the expression of S. All three are found almost exclusively in Blacks, which is an ethnic group being genotyped by many centers to supply blood for patients with SCD. Therefore, many of the current platforms include these SNPs in their final prediction of a phenotype. But there are other silencing mutations (eg, *JK*) that are not included because they are rare or found only in selected ethnic groups. To be able to have more accurate phenotypes predictions, future molecular tests will need to have these incorporated into the assay. The questions, however, are which ones, how many, and at what cost?

Automation

Two major goals that must be achieved before there is widespread use of red cell genotyping will be faster or automated assays and low cost per sample tested. Automated donor screening is already well accepted in the field of transfusion medicine so the acceptance of automated genotyping should not pose a problem. Presently, several automated platforms for DNA extraction exist that are capable of handling medium to large numbers of samples. Many of the microarray systems lend themselves well to being automated, and in fact, such systems are in development. However, some methods, such as the MALIDI-TOF-MS, are expensive and may never be a player in the blood bank market. Thus, the question must be asked: Will every hospital and blood center have the capabilities for rapid genotyping or will this type of testing be concentrated in large regional centers that have 24-hour capabilities and the needed molecular expertise?

The answer to this question will be, in part, dependent on how cost-effective the automated system is. Will the throughput be sufficient in a hospital or small blood center to warrant the high cost of the equipment? Will the reagent costs continue to rise as we have seen for the serologic reagents or will there be sufficient competition in the market to lower the cost per sample. As discussed earlier, there have been reports that existing methods are cost-effective and this should improve in the future. But a secondary force in determining reagent costs may be the existence of purchasing groups that, if they choose to pursue this route, may also help keep the cost of genotyping reasonable.

DATA MANAGEMENT

Assuming that automation will greatly enhance the numbers that can be genotyped daily and at a reasonable price, what is the next big challenge? It has to be data management. Interfaces will be needed between the instruments generating the data and the computers storing donor or patients' records, which will not be trivial because there are many different software systems used by hospitals and blood centers. Presently, there are blood centers performing microarray genotyping that easily generate 15,000 to 20,000 data points per month and there is much hands-on time involved in data review and management. With the implementation of the universal blood donor labeling (ie, ISBT 128 [International Society of Blood Transfusion]), it may be possible to bar code the sample from DNA extraction to end result. This advancement would greatly reduce manual entry errors that are common today.

Future Impact

Clearly, for selected populations, providing genotyped matched donors is not only desirable but is feasible. A study by Klapper and colleagues[32] showed that even with a limited donor pool, matching for Rh, Kell, Duffy Kidd, and MNSs could be achieved at least 50% of the time. Genotyping will probably not replace compatibility testing in the near future because the necessary donor pool is not yet available. But it certainly will be a strong adjunct, especially in patients where no serologic compatible blood can be found.

In 2009, a target of 100,000 HEA genotyped donors was achieved (G. Hashmi, personal communication, 2009), whereas more than 10,000 were genotyped in Canada.[14] As the donor base grows, we will be better able to provide genotyped matched blood including rare donor units. Already, the impact of wide-scale genotyping has had a positive effect on the American Rare Donor Program (ARDP). In the past, orders for Jo(a-) and Hy negative units have often gone unfilled; however, because of the availability of genotyped donors all such orders were met in 2009 (2009 ARDP Advisory Committee Report, unpublished data, 2009). It is interesting to speculate just what may be considered a rare donor once hundreds of thousands and even millions of donors have been genotyped. Having Lu(b-), Kp(b-), U negative, and so forth liquid on the shelf may be the future reality for the blood bank. But more importantly, is the fact that genotyping will provide better patient care for those needing chronic transfusion.

SUMMARY

A variety of molecular methods are currently being used for SNP typing and are amenable to red cell blood group typing. However, it is difficult to predict which will predominate and where the field of immunohematology might be even in as short a period as 10 years from now. The blending and evolution of molecular methods will certainly advance the use of red cell genotyping. This advancement, in combination with automation, will make large-scale screening a cost-effective reality. And in the era of personalized medicine it may not be so bizarre as to believe that all patients requiring transfusion will be genotyped for blood group antigens and donor units will be chosen based on a genotype match rather than a serologic crossmatch.

REFERENCES

1. Garratty G, Reid M, Westhoff C, editors. Proceedings of a workshop on molecular methods in immunohematology. Transfusion 2007;47(Suppl 1):S1–100S.
2. Moulds JM, Castilho L, Hashmi G, et al. Standards for molecular testing for red cell, platelet, and neutrophil antigens. 1st edition. Bethesda (MD): AABB; 2008.
3. Daniels G, Castilho L, Flegel WA, et al. International Society of Blood Transfusion committee on terminology for red cell surface antigens: Macao report. Vox Sang 2009;96:153–6.
4. Wagner FF, Bittne J, Doscher A, et al. Mid-throughput blood group phenotype prediction by pooled capillary electrophoresis. Transfusion 2008;48:1169–73.
5. Wu YY, Csako G. Rapid and/or high-throughput genotyping for red blood cell, platelet and leukocyte antigens, and forensic applications. Clin Chim Acta 2006;363:165–76.
6. Polin H, Danzer M, Proll J, et al. Introduction of a real-time based blood group genotyping approach. Vox Sang 2008;95:125–30.
7. Novaretti M, Dorlhiac-Llacer P, Chamone D, et al. Application of real-time PCR and melting curve analysis in rapid Diego blood group genotyping. Transfusion 2008;48(Suppl):195A.
8. Novaretti M, Ruiz A, Bonifacio SL, et al. Evaluation of PCR-ASP and real time PCR using fluorescent dye and melting curve analysis for yt(YT) blood group genotyping. Transfusion 2009;49(Suppl):134A.

9. Ansart-Pirenne H, Martin-Blanc S, Lepennec P-Y, et al. FY*X real-time polymerase chain reaction with melting curve analysis associated with a complete one-step real-time FY genotyping. Vox Sang 2007;92:142–7.

10. van Dronen J, Beckers EAM, Sintnocolaas K, et al. Rapid genotyping of blood group systems using the pyrosequencing technique. Vox Sang 2002; 83:104–5.

11. Beiboer SHW, Wieringa-Jelsma T, Maaskant-van Wijk PA, et al. Rapid genotyping of blood group antigens by multiplex polymerase chain reaction and DNA microarray hybridization. Transfusion 2005;45:667–79.

12. Hashmi G, Shariff T, Seul M, et al. A flexible array format for large-scale, rapid blood group DNA typing. Transfusion 2005;45:680–8.

13. Hashmi G, Shariff T, Zhang Y, et al. Determination of 24 minor red blood cell antigens for more than 2000 blood donors by high-throughput DNA analysis. Transfusion 2007;47:736–47.

14. Perreault J, Lavoie J, Painchaud P, et al. Set-up and routine use of a database of 10,555 genotyped blood donors to facilitate the screening of compatible blood components for alloimmunized patients. Vox Sang 2009;97:61–8.

15. Denomme GA, Van Oene M. High-throughput multiplex single-nucleotide polymorphism analysis for red cell and platelet antigen genotypes. Transfusion 2009;45:660–6.

16. Veldhuisen B, van der Schoot CE, De Haas M, et al. Blood group genotyping: from patient to high through-put donor screening. Vox Sang 2009;97: 198–206.

17. Karpasitou K, Drago F, Crespiatico L, et al. Blood group genotyping for Jk^a/Jk^b, Fy^a/Fy^b, S/s, Kp^a/Kp^b, Js^a/Js^b, Co^a/Cob, and Lu^a/Lu^b with microarray beads. Transfusion 2008;48:505–12.

18. Hopp K, Weber K, Bellissimo D, et al. Development of a new blood group genotyping platform using nanofluidic PCR. Transfusion 2008;48(Suppl):23A.

19. Hopp K, Weber K, Bellissimo D, et al. High-throughput red blood cell antigen genotyping using a nanofluidic real-time PCR polymerase chain reaction platform. Transfusion 2010;50(1):40–6.

20. Garritsen HSP, Fan AX-C, Lenz D, et al. Molecular diagnostics in transfusion medicine: In capillary, on a chip, in silico, or in flight. Transfus Med Hemother 2009;36:181–7.

21. Grill S, Banzola I, Li Y, et al. High throughput non-invasive determination of fetal rhesus D status using automated extraction of cell-free fetal DNA in maternal plasma and mass spectrometry. Arch Immunol Ther Exp 2009;279:533–7.

22. Ferri G, Bini C, Ceccardi S, et al. ABO genotyping by minisequencing analysis. Transfusion 2004;44:943–4.

23. Palacajornsuk P, Halter C, Isakova V, et al. Detection of blood group genes using multiple SNaPshot method. Transfusion 2009;49:740–9.

24. Anstee DJ. Red cell genotyping and the future of pretransfusion testing. Blood 2009;114:248–56.

25. Castro O, Sandler SG, Houston-Yu P, et al. Predicting the effect of transfusing only phenotype matched RBCs to patients with sickle cell disease: theoretical and practical implications. Transfusion 2002;42:684–90.

26. Allen TI, Billingsley KL, Slaughter J, et al. Red cell genotyping: a cost effective approach to screening large numbers of donors. Transfusion 2009;49(Suppl):135A.

27. Abumuhor IA, Klapper EB, Smith LE. The value of maintaining special screened RBC inventory by molecular testing in a tertiary care hospital. Transfusion 2009; 49(Suppl):242A.

28. Aygun B, Padmanabhan S, Paley C. Clinical significance of RBC alloantibodies and autoantibodies in sickle cell patients who received transfusions. Transfusion 2002;42:37–43.
29. Vichinsky EP, Luban NLC, Wright E, et al. Prospective RBC phenotype matching in a stroke-prevention trial in sickle cell anemia: a multicenter transfusion trial. Transfusion 2001;41:1086–92.
30. Petz L, Garratty G. Immune hemolytic anemias. Philadelphia: Churchill Livingstone; 2004. p. 379.
31. Reesink HW, Engelfriet CP, Schennach H, et al. Donors with a rare pheno (geno) type. Vox Sang 2005;95:236–53.
32. Klapper E, Zhang Y, Figueroa P, et al. Toward extended phenotype matching: a new operational paradigm for the transfusion service. Transfusion 2009. [Epub ahead of print].

Noninvasive Fetal Blood Grouping: Present and Future

Geoff Daniels, PhD, FRCPath*, Kirstin Finning, PhD, Pete Martin

KEYWORDS
- Noninvasive prenatal diagnosis • Fee fetal DNA
- Blood groups • Rh • Genotyping

Hemolytic disease of the fetus and newborn (HDFN) is caused by immunoglobulin (Ig)G antibodies to red cell surface antigens crossing the placenta and facilitating the immune destruction of fetal red cells or erythroid progenitors. The most common culprit antibody is directed to the D (RH1) blood group antigen of the Rh system. The reason for testing for fetal D phenotype in pregnant women with anti-D is to assist in the management of pregnancy. If the fetus is D-positive, appropriate management of a pregnancy at risk from HDFN can be arranged. If the fetus is D-negative, then it is not at risk, and no unnecessary interventions are required. Obtaining fetal red cells for serologic testing is a difficult and risky procedure, but cloning of the Rh genes in early 1990s[1–3] and the subsequent elucidation of the molecular bases to the D polymorphism[4,5] made it possible to predict D phenotype from the genotype obtained from fetal DNA. This now can be done with a high degree of accuracy. Fetal typing from DNA has been provided as a service in England since 1994. Initially the source of this fetal DNA was amniocytes or chorionic villi, but the procedures for obtaining these materials are expensive, invasive, and present a risk to the fetus. Amniocentesis is associated with a 0.5% to 1% risk of spontaneous abortion.[6] In addition, amniocentesis is associated with a 17% risk of transplacental hemorrhage,[7] which, if the fetus were D-positive, could boost the maternal anti-D, enhancing the risk of severe HDFN.

MATERNAL PLASMA AS A SOURCE OF FETAL DNA
Detection of Fetal DNA in Maternal Plasma

When Lo and colleagues[8] found fetal Y-chromosome sequence in the plasma of pregnant women bearing male fetuses, the implications for prenatal diagnostics without the requirement for invasive procedures were obvious. The main complication is that a very low concentration of fetal DNA is present in the maternal plasma. Lo and

International Blood Group Reference Laboratory, Bristol Institute for Transfusion Sciences, NHS Blood and Transplant, North Bristol Park, Northway, Filton, Bristol BS34 7QH, UK
* Corresponding author.
E-mail address: geoff.daniels@nhsbt.nhs.uk

Clin Lab Med 30 (2010) 431–442
doi:10.1016/j.cll.2010.02.006
0272-2712/10/$ – see front matter © 2010 Elsevier Inc. All rights reserved.

colleagues[9] used quantitative real-time polymerase chain reaction (PCR) analysis on *SRY* and β-globin gene sequences in pregnant women with a male fetus to show that fetal DNA represents about 3% (mean 25 genome equivalents/mL, range 3 to 69) of cell-free DNA in maternal plasma during the first trimester of pregnancy, rising to about 6% (mean 292 genome equivalents/mL, range 77 to 769) in the third trimester. Higher levels, up to 10%, have been found in other studies.[10,11] Free fetal DNA has been detected as early as 4 weeks' gestation.[12] Cell-free DNA in plasma of pregnant women consists of longer fragments than in nonpregnant women, whereas fetal fragments are much shorter than maternal fragments, with most of the fetally derived DNA molecules less than 0.3 kilobase (kb) in length.[13,14] Although enrichment of fetal DNA can be achieved by exploiting this differences in fragment size between fetal and maternal DNA, complete separation has not proved possible. Consequently, the only diagnostic tests on free fetal DNA in maternal plasma that are used routinely are those where the target gene is not present in the mother. These are fetal sexing by detection of a Y-borne gene and fetal blood grouping in women whose red cells lack the corresponding antigen.

Fetal DNA is cleared rapidly from the maternal plasma following delivery, with a mean half-life of 16 minutes following Caesarean section,[15] but clearance may take longer following labor, possibly to as much as 2 weeks.[16]

The high turnover of fetal DNA in maternal plasma, demonstrated by its rapid disappearance following delivery, suggests that fetal DNA is liberated continuously into the maternal circulation in large quantities.[15] The principal source of the fetal DNA is the placenta: normal levels of free fetal DNA were detected in anembryonic pregnancies with a placenta but with no fetus.[17] Villous trophoblasts within the fetal compartment of the placenta are released into the maternal blood via the feto–maternal interface and destroyed rapidly by the maternal immune system.[18,19] In addition, apoptosis in the villous trophoblasts in situ might lead to release of DNA into the maternal circulation.[20]

Does Fetal DNA Persist in the Maternal Plasma After Delivery?

Microchimerism, the engraftment of fetal cells in maternal lymphoid organs or bone marrow, leads to the persistence of very small numbers of nucleated cells in the mother's circulation many years after the pregnancy.[21] In 2002, Invernizzi and colleagues[22] detected Y-chromosome-specific sequences in plasma from 22% of healthy women with sons, in some cases many years after their last male pregnancy. Lambert and colleagues[23] found that DNA from previous pregnancies could be detected in DNA prepared following gentle centrifugation (400 g) of maternal plasma, but it was removed by passing the plasma through a 0.45 μm filter. This indicates that the DNA detected from previous pregnancies originates from cellular material, rather than free DNA in the plasma. Chiu and colleagues[24] recommend that if filtration is not employed, plasma should be microcentrifuged for 10 minutes at full speed (approximately 16 000 g) to remove all cellular material after the initial plasma separation.

PREDICTION OF D PHENOTYPE FROM FETAL DNA
The D Polymorphism

The antigens of the Rh system are encoded by *RHD* and *RHCE*, a pair of paralogous genes on chromosome 1. Each gene has 10 exons, and they share 94% sequence identity. They produce homologous proteins of 417 amino acids that are palmitoylated but not glycosylated. The proteins traverse the red cell membrane 12 times, with both termini in the cytosol and six extracellular loops, the potential sites for antigen activity.[25]

In Caucasians, where the frequency of D-negative phenotype is around 15%,[25] almost all D-negative individuals are homozygous for a deletion of the whole of *RHD*

(**Fig. 1**).[5] D-positive individuals may have one or two copies of *RHD*. The D-negative phenotype, therefore, almost always results from an absence of the RhD protein from the red cell membrane, although the RhCcEe protein is almost universally present.

In black Africans, where the frequency of D-negative phenotype is only about 5%,[25] the situation is different. Only 18% of D-negative black Africans are homozygous for an *RHD* deletion. Sixty-six percent of D-negative black Africans have an inactive *RHD* gene, called *RHDΨ*, which has a 37bp duplication in exon 4 and a nonsense mutation in exon 6, converting a tyrosine codon to a translation stop codon.[26] In addition, about 15% of D-negative black Africans have a hybrid gene, *RHD-CE-D^s*, that contains exons 1, 2, and 8 to10 from *RHD*, but exons 4 to 7 from *RHCE*; exon 3 may either be entirely or partly from *RHD* (see **Fig. 1**).[27–29] Neither *RHDΨ* nor *RHD-CE-D^s* produces any epitopes of D.

In eastern Asia, the D-negative phenotype is rare, with only about 2 in 1000 Chinese and Japanese being truly D-negative. Most of these are homozygous for a deletion of *RHD*, although *RHD-CE-D* hybrid genes are also present.[30]

There are numerous variants of the D antigen, recognized by absence of some or many D epitopes or weakness of expression of D.[25,31,32] In some cases, individuals with variant D antigens, if alloimmunized by normal D-positive red cells, can make antibodies to the D epitopes they lack from their own red cells. D-variant antigens result either from single nucleotide changes in *RHD* encoding amino acid substitutions or from hybrid Rh genes comprising sequences derived from both *RHD* and *RHCE* (see **Fig. 1**). A variant present in about 0.1% to 0.2% of Japanese and Chinese is DEL, in which the red cells appear to be D-negative by usual serologic methods, but D antigen is detectable by adsorption/elution techniques. DEL usually results from a synonymous mutation in the last (3′) nucleotide of exon 9 (1227G>A), which causes alternative splicing of the mRNA, with loss of exon 9, and so depletion of RhD protein.[30,33]

Fetal D Testing in Alloimmunized (High-risk) Pregnant Women

DNA usually is isolated from maternal plasma by centrifugation of EDTA-anticoagulated blood to remove the plasma, followed either by a second centrifugation at high speed or by filtration through a 0.2 μm filter, to remove all cellular material, which

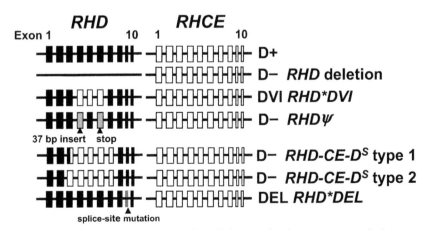

Fig. 1. Diagram of the Rh genes, *RHD* and *RHCE*, in seven haplotypes, one producing normal D (D+), one producing a variant (partial) D (DVI), one producing a very weak D that is not detectable by agglutination tests (DEL), and three producing no D (D–). Black boxes, *RHD* exons; white boxes, *RHCE* exons; gray boxes, mutated exons.

could originate from a previous pregnancy.[24] These procedures should take place as soon as possible after phlebotomy, to prevent breakdown of leucocytes and an increase in the proportion of maternal DNA.

Almost all laboratories performing fetal D typing on fetal DNA in maternal plasma employ real-time quantitative PCR (RQPCR) technology with Taqman chemistry.[34–36] The main advantages of RQPCR over conventional PCR are that it is quantitative, making it easy to distinguish fetal and maternal contributions, and the amplification and analysis takes place in closed tubes, reducing the risks of contamination.

Although amplification of a single region of *RHD* will provide a correct phenotype prediction in most cases, most protocols involve amplification of two or three exons to avoid obtaining false results with the more common variants of RHD. It is important that false positives do not result from the presence of the inactive African genes *RHDΨ* and *RHD-CE-D^s*. *RHDΨ* contains several single nucleotide polymorphisms (SNPs) in exons 4 and 5, and a negative result can be achieved by the use of primers or probes specific for the common sequence.[26,37] Amplification of any *RHD* sequence within exons 4 to 7 will give a correct negative result with *RHD-CE-D^s*. Many laboratories include an amplification of *RHD* exon 7 or exon 10. Exon 7 appears to provide a higher affinity reaction than exon 10.[38,39] Methods that employ amplification of exons 7 and 10 alone are not suitable for testing any population containing people of African origin, as they will give false-positive results when the fetus has *RHDΨ*. In addition, when the mother has *RHDΨ*, the very strongly positive reaction given by the maternal DNA will prevent identification of an active fetal *RHD*.

Matrix-assisted laser desorption ionization time of flight (MALDI-TOF) could be the technology of the future for fetal D typing. It would permit a large number of loci to be analyzed simultaneously, enhancing detection of fetal variant *RHD* genes, and allow for the incorporation of a panel of fetal markers to control for the presence of fetal DNA in D-negative female fetuses.[40] In one series of analyses with this technology for fetal *RHD* exon 7 on 178 clinical samples, 96.1% accuracy was obtained.[41]

Several reviews list most of the published studies on noninvasive fetal D testing.[42–45] A meta-analysis published in 2006 by Geifman-Holtzman and colleagues[43] analyzed 37 publications describing 44 protocols for fetal D testing from DNA in maternal blood. Their overall conclusion was accuracy of 94.8%, when excluding the small studies and excluding samples for absence of DNA or lack of Rh confirmation. In reality, the level of accuracy is much higher than this in laboratories providing a routine service. At the International Blood Group Reference Laboratory (IBGRL) in Bristol, United Kingdom, the authors have provided a noninvasive fetal *RHD* genotyping service since 2001 and tested about 1600 pregnancies. As far as the authors can ascertain only six erroneous results have been reported (two false-negative and four false-positive, two of which were from frozen plasma that could have been contaminated at source) (**Table 1**). Had amniocentesis been used to obtain fetal DNA for these tests, those errors might have been avoided, but one can estimate that between 8 and 16 of the fetuses would have been lost, and antibody levels would have been boosted in over 100 of the pregnant women.

The routine fetal RHD genotyping service in England is provided by the IBGRL (part of National Health Service Blood and Transplant) for alloimmunized pregnant D-negative women who require noninvasive monitoring and potentially intrauterine transfusions if they are carrying a D-positive fetus. This includes mothers with a previous history of fetal or neonatal hemolysis regardless of current anti-D level and those with a significant level of anti-D, usually defined as at least 4 IU/mL.

| Table 1 |
| Results of fetal blood grouping tests performed on free fetal DNA in maternal plasma at the IBGRL, United Kingdom, from 2002 to December 2009 ||||

Test	Number Tested	False Positive	False Negative
D	1609	4	2
C	19	0	0
c	309	0	0
E	316	0	0
K	554	1	1

Several similar services are provided around Europe,[36] but almost no noninvasive fetal D testing is performed in North America, although at least one service is provided in the United States.[46]

A fetal D typing method was designed specifically for a Chinese population and detected the *RHD*DEL* (1227G>A) allele.[47] From fetal tests on 78 D-negative Chinese women, 74 provided a result concordant with the serology: 60 D-positive, 10 D-negative, and 4 apparent D-negative, but with *RHD*DEL*.

One potential source of error is a previous transplant in the mother. Tests on DNA isolated from the plasma of a D-negative pregnant woman predicted a D-positive male fetus, whereas DNA isolated from amniocytes gave a D-negative result. The woman, who had received a kidney transplant from a D-positive male, delivered a D-negative girl.[48]

The Problem of Including Internal Controls

A problem in all tests on fetal DNA derived from maternal plasma arises from the large quantity of maternal DNA present in the DNA preparation, complicating the inclusion of satisfactory internal controls to test for successful amplification of fetal DNA. Without a control, an apparent D-negative result could arise from the presence of insufficient fetal DNA. One control that is used commonly is amplification of the Y-linked gene *SRY*, but this is only effective as a control when the fetus is male. When a result suggesting a D-negative female fetus is obtained, some laboratories have incorporated tests for a selection of polymorphisms that involve insertion or deletion of DNA sequence, in an attempt to obtain a positive result derived from fetal, but not maternal, DNA.[49] Short tandem repeats also may be employed in a similar way.[50,51] These methods have several drawbacks:

The tests are not true internal controls, as it is not possible to incorporate them as part of a multiplex with the *RHD* amplification.

They are often not informative unless a large number of polymorphisms are employed.

They are very labor-intensive, making the test time consuming and expensive.

They could give a false sense of security, as the test for the polymorphism may be more sensitive than the test for *RHD*.

Another potential method for introducing a control for the presence of fetal DNA in the presence of maternal DNA involves the exploitation of epigenetics: methylation of the cytosines of the dinucleotides of CpG islands in the 5′ region of certain genes in tissues where they are transcriptionally inactive. *RASSF1A* is a tumor suppressor gene in which the promoter is hypermethylated in fetal DNA and hypomethylated in maternal DNA.[52]

Treatment of DNA with the methylation-sensitive restriction enzyme *Bst*U1 results in digestion of an *RASSF1A* promoter sequence derived from maternal DNA, but not from fetal DNA, which originates from the placenta. The undigested sequences then could be detected by RQPCR in a multiplex with the test for *RHD*. This has potential for providing a suitable control, but difficulties can arise from incomplete digestion. So far there has only been one report of this technology being included into a diagnostic test, although it was not incorporated into the test as an internal control.[53]

Incorporation of reactions to housekeeping genes, such as *CCR5*, β-globin (*HBB*), β-actin (*ACTB*), or albumin (*ALB*), demonstrates that amplification has occurred, but will amplify fragments from both maternal and fetal DNA and so provide no control for the presence of adequate fetal DNA. When quantitative PCR is used, amplification of a housekeeping gene gives an estimate of the total amount of DNA present. If too much is detected, this probably arises from an excess of maternal DNA derived from cellular lysis before the plasma is removed, which could compromise the sensitivity of fetal DNA detection. The practice in IBGRL is to process the maternal blood within 48 hours of venepuncture. Spiking of the plasma with mouse DNA, maize DNA, or *Escherichia coli* plasmid, followed by specific detection, provides a control for sensitivity of the test.[54–56]

Simulation of DNA derived from a pregnant woman prepared by spiking DNA from an adult with a small quantity human DNA that is not of fetal origin is not suitable for use in quality control or validation of fetal genotyping tests, because fetal DNA fragments are much shorter than maternal fragments.[13,14]

Fetal Testing to Ascertain the Requirement for Antenatal Anti-D Immunoglobulin Prophylaxis

Although anti-D immunoglobulin prophylaxis given following the birth of a D-positive baby eliminated most anti-D alloimmunization, a low level of immunization still occurred during the pregnancy. In 1978, a clinical trial showed that giving 1500 IU of anti-D immunoglobulin at 28 and 34 weeks' gestation reduced immunization during pregnancy from 1.8% to 0.14%.[57] It is now policy in many countries to offer one or two doses of anti-D immunoglobulin antenatally, around 28 weeks' gestation. In a predominantly Caucasian population, however, about 38% of these women would be carrying a D-negative fetus and receive this treatment unnecessarily.[25] So far, lack of a safe and reliable technique of sufficiently high-throughput for routine fetal *RHD* genotyping has meant that to protect all D-negative women, those with a D-negative fetus also receive prophylaxis.

Two sets of trials have been described employing high-throughput methods, including robotic isolation of plasma DNA and RQPCR technology, with the potential for testing the fetal D type for all D-negative pregnant women. In the Netherlands, 2359 samples taken at 30 weeks' gestation were tested for *RHD* exon 7.[58] In the 1257 cases in which molecular results could be compared with serologic results, three false-negative results and five false-positive results were obtained, giving a diagnostic accuracy of 99.4%. In the United Kingdom, Finning and colleagues[59] analyzed *RHD* exons 5 (negative with *RHDΨ*) and 7 (positive with *RHDΨ*) from maternal plasma. CCR5 was included as an amplification control. A correct fetal D phenotype was predicted by the genotyping tests in 95.7% of 1869 pregnancies in which a serologic D phenotype was obtained from the cord blood samples. In 3.4% of cases, results were either unobtainable or inconclusive. In 0.75% (14 samples) a false-positive result was obtained, probably because of unexpressed or weakly expressed fetal *RHD* genes. In only three samples (0.16%) were false-negative results obtained. It is these false-negatives that cause most concern, as in a diagnostic setting, anti-D immunoglobulin prophylaxis would have been withheld, with a resultant risk of immunization. In all three cases, however, the blood samples had been delayed in transport before plasma isolation and would not have been accepted for diagnostic testing. If the results of the UK trials had been applied as a guide to treatment, only 2% of the women would have received anti-D immunoglobulin unnecessarily, compared with 38% without the genotyping.

A large validation study of over 1000 D-negative pregnant women in Germany showed 99.5% accuracy.[60] A similar level of accuracy was achieved in a French analysis of almost 900 pregnancies, but this study required retesting all negative results, and so would be uneconomical for screening D-negative pregnant women.[39]

There will be many advantages to performing fetal D testing of all D-negative pregnant women. Most importantly, it eliminates unnecessary treatment of pregnant women with blood products and the associated inconvenience, discomfort, and perceived risks of infection from pooled donor blood products that such injections entail. Blood services world-wide are spending increasing sums of money to ensure the safety of the blood supply. Fetal *RHD* screening provides a way of significantly reducing the quantity of blood products given routinely to pregnant women. In addition, there will be no requirement to give anti-D immunoglobulin antenatally to women with D-negative fetuses after potential sensitizing events such as amniocentesis or other trauma. Although anti-D immunoglobulin can be considered a safe product, with millions of doses having been given with no infectious complications, it should be noted that hundreds of women were infected with hepatitis C virus transmitted by anti-D immunoglobulin in Ireland from 1977 to 1978.[61] A D-negative woman with severe inherited factor XI deficiency produced an inhibitor antibody, induced by factor XI in anti-D immunoglobulin.[62] Such an event would be extremely rare, but it is a reminder that anti-D immunoglobulin contains more than just anti-D. Clinicians or midwives can advise on the risks and benefits of receiving anti-D immunoglobulin. Anti-D immunoglobulin is in short supply, and it is produced from plasma of volunteers who have been immunized with D-positive red cells, so there is an ethical issue about immunizing people with blood products to produce a drug that might be rendered unnecessary in a substantial portion of D-negative pregnant women if a test for fetal D type were available. Furthermore, the cost of the test might be less than the cost of anti-D immunoglobulin, but no thorough economic evaluation has been published. If the test proved accurate enough, there would be no need to test cord red cells serologically for D.

FETAL GENOTYPING FOR OTHER BLOOD GROUPS

After anti-D, the next most common causes of HDFN are anti-c (anti-RH4) of the Rh system and anti-K (anti-KEL1) of the Kell system.[25] Antibodies to the Rh antigens C (RH2) and E (RH3) also occasionally cause severe HDFN. The molecular background to the c/C polymorphism is complex, but is basically a 307C>T SNP in exon 2 of *RHCE* encoding Pro103Ser in the second extracellular loop of the RhCcEe protein.[63] C307 can be detected to recognize the presence of an *RHCE*c* allele. The situation for C is more complicated, as the sequences of exon 2 of *RHCE*C* and *RHD* are identical making specific amplification of *RHCE*C* impossible in D-positives. *RHCE*C* has a 109bp insert in intron 2 that is not present in *RHCE*c* or *RHD*, however, and this can be used for C typing.[64] The e/E polymorphism results from a 676G>C SNP in exon 5 of *RHCE* encoding Ala226Pro in the fourth extracellular loop of the protein,[63] so typing for E involves detection of C676. The k/K polymorphism results from a 578C>T SNP in exon 6 of *KEL* encoding Thr193Met.[65]

There are only a few published reports of noninvasive fetal genotyping for C, c, and E.[56,66–69] All involve RQPCR with allele-specific primers or probes. The genotyping results, compared with serologic determinations following birth, show 100% accuracy. **Table 1** shows the results obtained at IBGRL, Bristol, United Kingdom since the authors began testing for C, c, E, K.

K typing presents more of a problem. Finning and colleagues[67] were unable to obtain a satisfactory level of specificity by conventional RQPCR methods owing to mispriming of the K (KEL*1) allele-specific primer on the k (KEL*2) allele. This was overcome, with a sacrifice of reduced sensitivity, by employing locked nucleic acids (LNAs) and the introduction of a mismatch into the allele-specific primer. LNAs are nucleic acid analogs, which lock the structure into a rigid bicyclic formation.[70] Oligonucleotides that contain LNAs have exceptionally high affinity to complementary DNA strands and excellent mismatch discrimination. At IBGRL, the authors have had one false-negative and one false-positive result from testing over 500 pregnancies (see **Table 1**). The false-negative result was obtained in a sample taken at 17 weeks' gestation that had a particularly low yield of total DNA. It is now a recommendation in England that K testing should not be performed before 20 weeks' gestation and that a K-negative result obtained before 28 weeks should be followed up with a repeat test at or after 28 weeks.

In one set of tests, fetal K detection by MALDI-TOF mass spectrometry-based single allele-based extension reaction, 94% accuracy was obtained.[71]

Most K antibodies are stimulated by blood transfusion, rather than pregnancy.[72] Consequently, the partners of many women with anti-K are K-negative, indicating a K-negative fetus. It is valuable, therefore, to test the father for K before making the decision to carry out fetal testing.

QUALITY ASSURANCE

As an increasing number of laboratories internationally are introducing noninvasive fetal blood group testing, it is important that their performances are monitored through external quality assurance (EQA) schemes. The International Society of Blood Transfusion (ISBT) has organized three international workshops in molecular blood group genotyping.[34–36] In the most recent workshop (2008), two plasma samples from pregnant D-negative women, one with a D-positive and one with a D-negative fetus, were distributed to 17 laboratories (14 from Europe, one each from Australia, Brazil, and China). From a total of 31 results submitted, 27 were correct, two were inconclusive, and two reported the D-positive fetus as D-negative (**Table 2**). All laboratories employed RQPCR.[36]

A workshop on extraction of fetal DNA from maternal plasma demonstrated that the highest yield was obtained by the QIAamp DSP virus kit (Qiagen, Valencia, CA, USA).[73]

Table 2
Plasma fetal RHD typing results from ISBT workshop 2008 (17 laboratories received samples)

Fetal D Type	Correct	Incorrect	Inconclusive	No Results Reported
D-negative	14	0	1	2
D-positive	13	2	1	1

From Daniels G, van der Schoot CE, Gassner C, et al. Report of the Third International Workshop on Molecular Blood Group Genotyping. Vox Sang 2009;96:337–43. Available at: http://www.ibgrl.blood.co.uk. Accessed December 16, 2009.

SUMMARY

To date, the enormous promise of the application of free fetal DNA in maternal plasma to prenatal diagnostics mainly has been realized in fetal blood grouping and fetal sexing, though it is also applied to single gene disorders where it is currently restricted to disease-causing mutations not present in maternal genome, such as paternally inherited dominant disorders (eg, Huntington disease) and recessive diseases where the maternal and paternal mutations often differ (eg, cystic fibrosis).[74]

Fetal blood grouping often plays an important role in the avoidance of unnecessary procedures and is the standard of care in England for pregnant women with significant levels of anti-D. Because a reliable noninvasive test is available, it could be considered unethical to perform amniocenteses purely for fetal D typing. In the future, high-throughput fetal D typing will reduce wastage of anti-D immunoglobulin and avoid unnecessary treatment of pregnant women with blood products. As intellectual property rights have been granted for free fetal DNA testing worldwide, one can hope that progress in this field will not be hampered by financial and legal issues.

REFERENCES

1. Avent ND, Ridgwell K, Tanner MJA, et al. cDNA cloning of a 30 kDa erythrocyte membrane protein associated with Rh (Rhesus)-blood-group-antigen expression. Biochem J 1990;271:821–5.
2. Chérif-Zahar B, Bloy C, Le Van Kim C, et al. Molecular cloning and protein structure of a human blood group Rh polypeptide. Proc Natl Acad Sci U S A 1990;87: 6243–7.
3. Le Van Kim C, Mouro I, Chérif-Zahar B, et al. Molecular cloning and primary structure of the human blood group RhD polypeptide. Proc Natl Acad Sci U S A 1992; 89:10925–9.
4. Colin Y, Chérif-Zahar B, Le Van Kim C, et al. Genetic basis of the RhD-positive and RhD-negative blood group polymorphism as determined by Southern analysis. Blood 1991;78:2747–52.
5. Wagner FF, Flegel WA. *RHD* gene deletion occurred in the Rhesus box. Blood 2000;95:3662–8.
6. Wilson RD. Amniocentesis and chorionic villus sampling. Curr Opin Obstet Gynecol 2000;12:81–6.
7. Tabor A, Bang J, Nørgaard-Pedersen B. Feto-maternal haemorrhage associated with genetic amniocentesis: results of a randomized trial. Br J Obstet Gynaecol 1987;94:528–34.
8. Lo YM, Corbetta N, Chamberlain PF, et al. Presence of fetal DNA in maternal plasma and serum. Lancet 1997;350:485–7.
9. Lo YM, Tein MS, Lau TK, et al. Quantitative analysis of fetal DNA in maternal plasma and serum: implications for noninvasive prenatal diagnosis. Am J Hum Genet 1998;62:768–75.
10. van der Schoot CE, Tax GH, Rijnders RJ, et al. Prenatal typing of RH and Kell blood group system antigens: the edge of a watershed. Transfus Med Rev 2003;17:31–44.
11. Lun FM, Chiu RW, Chan KC, et al. Microfluidics digital PCR reveals a higher than expected fraction of fetal DNA in maternal plasma. Clin Chem 2008;10:1664–72.
12. Illanes S, Denbow M, Kailasam C, et al. Early detection of cell-free fetal DNA in maternal plasma. Early Hum Dev 2007;83:563–6.
13. Chan KC, Zhang J, Hui AB, et al. Size distribution of maternal and fetal DNA in maternal plasma. Clin Chem 2004;50:88–92.

14. Li Y, Zimmermann B, Rusterholz C, et al. Size separation of circulatory DNA in maternal plasma permits ready detection of fetal DNA polymorphisms. Clin Chem 2004;50:1002–11.
15. Lo YM, Zhanf J, Leung TN, et al. Rapid clearance of fetal DNA from maternal plasma. Am J Hum Genet 1999;64:218–24.
16. Hui L, Vaughan JI, Nelson M. Effect of labor on postpartum clearance of cell-free fetal DNA from the maternal circulation. Prenat Diagn 2008;28:304–8.
17. Alberry M, Maddocks D, Jones M, et al. Free fetal DNA in maternal plasma in anembryonic pregnancies: confirmation that the origin is the trophoblast. Prenat Diagn 2007;27:415–8.
18. Poon LL, Lo YM. Circulating fetal DNA in maternal plasma. Clin Chim Acta 2001; 313:151–5.
19. Bianchi DW. Circulating fetal DNA: its origin and diagnostic potential—a review. Placenta 2004;25(Suppl A):S93–101.
20. Levy R, Nelson DM. To be, or not to be, that is the question. Apoptosis in human trophoblast. Placenta 2000;21:1–13.
21. Bianchi DW, Zickwolf GK, Weil GJ, et al. Male fetal progenitor cells persist in maternal blood for as long as 27 years postpartum. Proc Natl Acad Sci U S A 1996;93:705–8.
22. Invernizzi P, Biondi ML, Battezzati PM, et al. Presence of fetal DNA in maternal plasma decades after pregnancy. Hum Genet 2002;110:587–91.
23. Lambert NC, Lo YM, Erickson TD, et al. Male microchimerism in healthy women and women with scleroderma: cells or circulating DNA? A quantitative answer. Blood 2002;100:2845–51.
24. Chiu RW, Poon LL, Lau TK, et al. Effects of blood-processing protocols on fetal and total DNA quantification in maternal plasma. Clin Chem 2001;9:1607–13.
25. Daniels G. Human blood groups. 2nd edition. Oxford: Blackwell Science; 2002.
26. Singleton BK, Green CA, Avent ND, et al. The presence of an RHD pseudogene containing a 37 base pair duplication and a nonsense mutation in most Africans with the Rh D-negative blood group phenotype. Blood 2000;95:12–8.
27. Faas BH, Beckers EA, Wildoer P, et al. Molecular background of VS and weak C expression in blacks. Transfusion 1997;37:38–44.
28. Daniels GL, Faas BH, Green CA, et al. The Rh VS and V blood group polymorphisms in Africans: a serological and molecular analysis. Transfusion 1998;38: 951–8.
29. Pham BN, Peyrard T, Juszczak G, et al. Heterogeneous molecular background of the weak C, VS+, hr^B, Hr^B phenotype in black persons. Transfusion 2009;49: 495–504.
30. Shao CP, Maas JH, Su YQ, et al. Molecular background of Rh D-positive, D-negative, Del and weak D phenotypes in Chinese. Vox Sang 2002;83:156–61.
31. Wagner FF, Gassner C, Müller TH, et al. Molecular basis of weak D phenotypes. Blood 1999;93:385–93.
32. List of D variants. Available at: http://rhesusbase.atspace.com. Accessed December 16, 2009.
33. Shao CP, Xiong X, Zhou YY. Multiple isoforms excluding normal RhD mRNA detected in Rh blood group D$_{el}$ phenotype with RHD 1227A allele. Transfus Apheresis Sci 2006;34:145–52.
34. Daniels G, van der Schoot CE, Olsson ML. Report of the first international workshop on molecular blood group genotyping. Vox Sang 2005;88:136–42.
35. Daniels G, van der Schoot E, Olsson ML. Report of the Second International Workshop on molecular blood group genotyping. Vox Sang 2007;93:83–8.

36. Daniels G, van der Schoot CE, Gassner C, et al. Report of the Third International Workshop on molecular blood group genotyping. Vox Sang 2009;96:337–43. Available at: http://ibgrl.blood.co.uk. Accessed December 16, 2009.
37. Finning K, Martin P, Daniels G. The use of maternal plasma for prenatal RhD blood group genotyping. In: Bugert P, editor, DNA and RNA profiling in human blood: methods and protocols, vol. 496. New York: Humana Press; 2009. p. 143–57.
38. Aubin JT, Le Van Kim C, Mouro I, et al. Specificity and sensitivity of RHD genotyping methods by PCR-based DNA amplification. Br J Haematol 1997;98:356–64.
39. Rouillac-Le Sciellour C, Puillandre P, Gillot R, et al. Large-scale prediagnosis study of fetal *RHD* genotyping by PCR on plasma DNA from RhD-negative pregnant women. Mol Diagn 2004;8:23–31.
40. van der Schoot CE, Hahn S, Chitty LS. Non-invasive pre-natal diagnosis and determination of fetal Rh status. Semin Fetal Neonatal Med 2008;13:63–8.
41. Grill S, Banzola I, Ying L, et al. High throughput non-invasive determination of foetal Rhesus D status using automated extraction of cell-free foetal DNA in maternal plasma and mass spectometry. Arch Gynecol Obstet 2009;279:533–7.
42. Daniels G, Finning K, Martin P, et al. Fetal blood group genotyping from DNA from maternal plasma: an important advance in the management and prevention of haemolytic disease of the fetus and newborn. Vox Sang 2004;87:225–32.
43. Geifman-Holtzman O, Grotegut CA, Gaughan JP. Diagnostic accuracy of noninvasive fetal genotyping from maternal blood – a meta analysis. Am J Obstet Gynecol 2006;195:1163–73.
44. Daniels G, Finning K, Martin P, et al. Non-invasive prenatal diagnosis of fetal blood group phenotypes: current practice and future prospects. Prenat Diagn 2009;29:101–7.
45. Maddocks DG, Alberry MS, Attilakos G, et al. The SAFE project: towards noninvasive prenatal diagnosis. Biochem Soc Trans 2009;37:460–5.
46. Brochure from Lenetix. Available at: http://www.lenetix.com. Accessed December 16, 2009.
47. Wang XD, Wang BL, Ye SL, et al. Non-invasive fetal *RHD* genotyping via real-time PCR of foetal DNA from Chinese RhD-negative maternal plasma. Eur J Clin Invest 2009;39:607–17.
48. Minon JM, Semterre JM, Schaaps JP, et al. An unusual false positive fetal RHD typing result using DNA derived from maternal plasma from a solid organ recipient. Transfusion 2006;46:1454.
49. Page-Christiaens GC, Bossers B, van der Schoot CE, et al. Use of bi-allelic insertion/deletion polymorphisms as a positive control in maternal blood. First clinical experience. Ann N Y Acad Sci 2006;1075:123–9.
50. Pertl B, Pieber D, Panzitt T, et al. RhD genotyping by quantitative fluorescent polymerase chain reaction: a new approach. Br J Obstet Gynaecol 2000;107:1498–502.
51. Liu FM, Wang XY, Feng X, et al. Feasibility study of using fetal DNA in maternal plasma for noninvasive prenatal diagnosis. Acta Obstet Gynecol Scand 2007; 86:535–41.
52. Chan KC, Ding C, Gerovassili A, et al. Hypermethylated *RASSF1A* in maternal plasma: a universal fetal DNA marker that improves the reliability of noninvasive prenatal diagnosis. Clin Chem 2006;52:2211–8.
53. Hyland CA, Gardener GJ, Davies H, et al. Evaluation of noninvasive prenatal *RHD* genotyping of the fetus. Med J Aust 2009;191:21–5.
54. Rouillac-Le Sciellour C, Sérazin V, Brossard Y, et al. Noninvasive fetal *RHD* genotyping from maternal plasma. Use of a new developed Free DNA Fetal Kit RhD®. Transfus Clin Biol 2007;14:572–7.

55. Costa JM, Giovangrandi Y, Ernault P, et al. Fetal *RHD* genotyping in maternal serum during the first trimester of pregnancy. Br J Haematol 2002;119:255–60.

56. Legler TJ, Lynen R, Maas JH, et al. Prediction of fetal Rh D and Rh CcEe phenotype from maternal plasma with real-time polymerase chain reaction. Transfus Apheresis Sci 2002;27:217–23.

57. Bowman JM, Chown B, Lewis M, et al. Rh immunization during pregnancy, antenatal prophylaxis. Can Med Assoc J 1978;118:623.

58. van der Schoot CE, Ait Soussan A, Koelewijn J, et al. Noninvasive antenatal *RHD* typing. Transfus Clin Biol 2006;13:53–7.

59. Finning K, Martin P, Summers J, et al. Effect of high-throughput RHD typing of fetal DNA in maternal plasma on use of anti-RhD immunoglobulin in RhD negative pregnant women: prospective feasibility study. Br Med J 2008;336:816–8.

60. Müller SP, Bartels I, Stein W, et al. The determination of the fetal D status from maternal plasma for decision making on Rh prophylaxis is feasible. Transfusion 2008;48:2292–301.

61. Kenny-Walsh E. Clinical outcomes after hepatitis C infection from contaminated anti-D immune globulin. N Engl J Med 1999;340:1228–33.

62. Zucker M, Zivelin A, Teitel J, et al. Induction of an inhibitor antibody to factor XI in a patient with severe inherited factor XI deficiency by Rh immune globulin. Blood 2008;111:1306–8.

63. Mouro I, Colin Y, Chérif-Zahar B, et al. Molecular genetic basis of the human Rhesus blood group system. Nat Genet 1993;5:62–5.

64. Poulter M, Kemp TJ, Carritt B. DNA-based Rhesus typing: simultaneous determination of RHC and RHD status using the polymerase chain reaction. Vox Sang 1996;70:164–8.

65. Lee S, Wu X, Reid M, et al. Molecular basis of the Kell (K1) phenotype. Blood 1995;85:912–6.

66. Hromadnikova I, Vechetova L, Vesela K, et al. Non-invasive fetal RHD and RHCE genotyping using real-time PCR testing of maternal plasma in RhD-negative pregnancies. J Histochem Cytochem 2005;53:301–5.

67. Finning K, Martin P, Summers J, et al. Fetal genotyping for the K (Kell) and Rh C, c, and E blood groups on cell-free fetal DNA from maternal plasma. Transfusion 2007;47:2126–33.

68. Orzińska A, Guz K, Brojer E, et al. Preliminary results with fetal Rhc examination in plasma of pregnant women with anti-c. Prenat Diagn 2008;28:335–7.

69. Geifman-Holtzman O, Grotegut CA, Gaughan JP, et al. Noninvasive fetal RhCE genotyping from maternal blood. BJOG 2009;116:144–51.

70. Petersen K, Vogel U, Rockenbauer E, et al. Short PNA molecular beacons for real-time PCR allelic discrimination of single nucleotide polymorphisms. Mol Cell Probes 2004;18:117–22.

71. Li Y, Finning K, Daniels G, et al. Noninvasive genotyping fetal Kell blood group (KEL1) using cell-free fetal DNA in maternal plasma by MALDI-TOF mass spectometry. Prenat Diagn 2008;28:203–8.

72. Klein HG, Anstee DJ. Blood transfusion in clinical medicine. 11th edition. Oxford: Blackwell; 2005.

73. Legler TJ, Liu Z, Mavrou A, et al. Workshop report on the extraction of foetal DNA from maternal plasma. Prenat Diagn 2007;27:824–9.

74. Wright CF, Chitty LS. Cell-free fetal DNA and RNA in maternal blood: implications for safer antenatal testing. BMJ 2009;339:161–4 (b2451).

Current and Future Cellular Transfusion Products

Monique P. Gelderman, PhD*, Jaroslav G. Vostal, MD, PhD

KEYWORDS

• Red cells • Platelets • Transfusion
• Novel transfusion products

Each year millions of life-saving and quality of life-enhancing blood components are collected and transfused. The cellular transfusion products, which include red blood cells (RBCs) and platelets, are collected and processed by approved methods to ensure their safety, purity, and potency. Novel transfusion products may be synthetic or may result from modifications to approved collection, processing, and storage procedures for existing cellular products and must be reviewed by the Food and Drug Administration (FDA) before being legally marketed in the United States. Manufacturers of novel transfusion products typically have performed in vitro studies, small Phase I and Phase 2 clinical trials, and larger Phase 3 trials to evaluate their products. For modified components, the extent of studies required depends, in part, on whether the novel RBC or platelet product is collected using methods that are significantly different from approved methods. Novel RBC products include RBCs collected in new storage bags or bags with new anticoagulants, RBCs derived from stem cells, RBCs subject to extended storage, and RBCs undergoing pathogen reduction procedures. Novel platelet products include pathogen-reduced platelets, extended-storage platelets and lyophilized platelets used for intravenous hemostasis, stem-cell derived platelets, and platelet products stored or derived in other ways that may influence product safety or quality. Artificial particles with platelet-like hemostatic functions also are being developed. Evaluation of these novel products involves testing to establish whether the product is safe, pure, and potent.

Current transfusion therapies and practices are the culmination of major scientific and technological advancements during the last 7 decades. Nevertheless, innovative technologies have the potential to improve blood and blood products. The FDA

The findings and conclusions in this manuscript have not been formally disseminated by the FDA and should not be construed to represent any Agency determination or policy.
Laboratory of Cellular Hematology, Division of Hematology, Office of Blood Research and Review, Center for Biologics Evaluation and Research, Food and Drug Administration, 1401 Rockville Pike, HFM-335, Rockville, MD 20852-1448, USA
* Corresponding author.
E-mail address: monique.gelderman-fuhrmann@fda.hhs.gov

regulates biologic products, including blood and blood products, to ensure that they are safe, pure, and potent. Thus, novel products that seek to further improve currently available products (eg, extending the shelf life) are evaluated by the FDA. In this article, we discuss certain novel products of potential interest in transfusion medicine that are described in the literature.

RBC TRANSFUSION PRODUCTS

RBCs are a life-saving therapeutic transfusion component. Approximately fifteen million RBCs units are collected and transfused in the United States each year[1] with the intent of providing increased capacity to deliver oxygen to tissues of patients who are anemic.

The FDA evaluates novel RBC products to ensure that they are safe, pure, and potent and at least equivalent to other RBC transfusion products already on the market. The FDA evaluation process relies, in part, on in vitro tests and on RBC recovery based on in vivo radiolabeling clinical studies. The in vitro tests characterize RBC morphology and biochemical status that include red cell shape, size, hemoglobin concentration, hemolysis, cell surface markers, glucose use rates, lactate production rates, ATP levels, and use rates. Some of these tests have been in use for decades while others have been recently developed and adapted. These tests do not include evaluation of oxygen-carrying capacity because, historically, it has been assumed that minor modifications to storage conditions do not alter the RBC ability to deliver oxygen. Extrapolation of in vitro tests results to predict the in vivo function of RBCs has had, over the years, only limited success. Highly abnormal tests are usually predictive of poor in vivo performance but normal or slightly abnormal in vitro tests may also be associated with decreased in vivo performance.

It is well accepted that the viability of a sample of stored red cells cannot be accurately predicted from any measurement made in vitro. Therefore, measurements of posttransfusion survival are necessary to assess potential new methods of collection and storage.[2] Because of the difficulty of extrapolating in vitro results to clinical performance the FDA has relied on in vivo studies as the gold standard for evaluation of RBC products. The in vivo test involves radiolabeling of autologous RBCs donated by a healthy volunteer and reinfusion of these cells into the same volunteer. The percentage of the RBCs recovered 24 hours after transfusion has been used to evaluate the quality of RBCs. This criterion for evaluating in vivo recovery of RBCs has evolved over time along with new procedures and technologies.

In 2008, the Blood Products Advisory Committee (BPAC) addressed the issue of RBC recovery. The BPAC supported (15 yes, 2 no) that radiolabeling studies for RBC recovery should be performed in at least two separate laboratories with a total of 20 to 24 healthy donors. The mean recovery at 24 hours for each unit should be greater than or equal to 75% with SD less than or equal to 9%; and the one-sided 95% lower confidence limit for the population proportion of successes greater than 70%.[3]

Recent studies have highlighted potential risks associated with RBCs stored for longer periods before transfusion. Two retrospective analyses indicated that transfusion of older RBCs to critically ill patients may lead to adverse events and ultimately death.[4,5] Prospective studies evaluating clinical outcomes of patients transfused with different aged RBCs are needed to determine if older RBCs may be detrimental for certain patient groups.[6,7] Several large prospective studies evaluating different clinical outcomes are being initiated in the United States (the Red Cell Storage Duration Study [RECESS]) and Canada (the Age of Red Cells in Premature Infants

[ARIPI]).[8,9] The results of these studies will help to determine if there is a correlation between the age of the transfused RBCs and the evaluated clinical outcomes.

Extension of RBC Shelf Life

Potential shortages of RBCs continues to be a concern. Liquid-stored RBCs maintain their viability and function for 42 days when stored in compliance with federal regulations and American Association of Blood Banks guidelines.[10,11] Some researchers have studied methods for extending RBC shelf life without compromising integrity and effectiveness. Other scientists have worked to develop a transfusion product with the same function as RBCs but processed by alternative means or generated from alternative sources. One group of researchers, for example, removed the oxygen from RBCs and subsequently maintained them under anaerobic conditions.[12] Storage under anaerobic conditions combined with metabolic rejuvenation extended the useful RBC shelf life to 12 weeks.[13] The results of a recent in vivo study by the same group indicated that anaerobic storage of RBCs stored in a novel additive solution may represent an improvement compared with conventionally stored RBCs.[14] These studies may help to address the need to increase RBC availability by allowing these products to be stored for longer periods.

"Universal Donor" RBCs

At present, investigators are looking at the possibility of producing RBC transfusion products that are "ageless" and with a "universal donor" quality. This may seem unattainable, but a substantial amount of research has already been published on ex vivo production of RBCs.[15–17] These investigators have explored the use of stem cells as a potential source of transfusable blood products. Researchers may use stem cells with reduced antigens to produce an RBC transfusion product with a "universal donor" quality. However, there are several different progenitor cell types that can become committed to either the erythroid or the platelet lineage. A few examples of potential progenitor cell types are bone marrow, cord blood, peripheral blood, and embryonic stem cells. Investigators using cord blood-derived CD34+ cells, for instance, have been successful in driving these cells into mature RBCs. The choice of progenitor cells is based on the likely degree of commitment to a given lineage as well as logistical, cost, and ethical considerations.

Creating "universal donor" RBCs using conventionally collected RBCs by enzymatic conversion of blood group A and B RBCs to blood group O also may be possible. However, clinical experience with enzyme-converted RBCs has shown that cross-match reactivity remains and thus additional in vitro and in vivo work in this area will be needed.[18]

Pathogen Reduction of RBCs

Currently, the FDA ensures blood safety by using a multilayered approach that includes screening donors for risk factors for infectious disease and testing blood for specific agents. This approach has worked well and dramatically reduced the incidence of transfusion-transmitted disease.

Occasionally pathogens are not detected by screening tests because organisms are present at levels that are below the assay's level of detection. Even with testing and donor deferral due to travel restrictions, it is estimated that the residual risk of a transfusion transmitted disease from transfusion products is in the order of 1 per 277, 000 for viral pathogens, 1 per 70,000 to 118,000 for bacterial agents, and 1 per 1,000,000 for protozoa.[19]

In addition, the potential exists for emergence of a new pathogen for which screening tests are not available. Pathogen reduction of blood components holds

liquid storage has been problematic. It has been difficult to preserve platelet ability to function as a cell and to participate in hemostatic events without causing unwanted thrombosis.

Another approach has been to engineer platelet-like agents from unrelated materials and attach either platelet proteins or peptides that can mimic some aspects of platelet function. Frequently, the peptides will bind activated platelets through the conformationally altered glycoprotein IIb/IIIa that binds fibrinogen.[42,43] Though these products could add to an already formed platelet plug, they will not function on their own. However, even if such products are unable to replicate the full range of platelet function, they still may be useful for specific clinical applications.

Stem Cell-Derived Platelets

Another method of platelet manufacture is to use pluripotent stem cells found in stem cell-enriched samples such as cord blood or peripheral stem cells.[44] The pluripotent cells in these cell populations can be directed toward development of megakaryocytes and, ultimately of platelets under the influence of cytokine cocktails.[45] A variety of logistical issues need to be addressed for large-scale production of stem cell-derived platelets for these types of products to become practical, including availability of the source material and lowering the cost of production.

Evaluation of Novel RBC and Platelet-Transfusion Products

The evaluation of novel cellular-transfusion products by manufacturers will depend on the issues raised by the specific product and how different it is from a currently approved product.[46] The FDA has issued a draft guidance on evaluating platelet products.[47] The FDA may hold workshops to assess the science related to novel products and to help develop standards. The FDA also may bring novel products for scientific discussion before the BPAC.

Typically, the product's characteristics are measured by in vitro tests, focusing on a variety of cellular responses such as aggregation- and agonist-induced shape change for platelets and responses to osmotic stress and oxygen-binding characterization for RBCs.[47] Manufacturers also compare novel products to platelet or RBC products collected by currently approved methods.

Large differences in the average responses of in vitro tests may predict significant differences in the clinical performance of the transfusion product.

There are several in vitro tests that have a defined endpoint required in the Code of Federal Regulations (eg, a pH value >6.2 at the end of the shelf life of a platelets product, which currently is 5 days),[48] or have become established industry standards. Products should meet statistically defined criteria for quality based on in vitro tests with a recognized endpoint. For example, in a recent draft guidance document on leukocyte-reduced RBCs, the FDA proposed that 95% of the products should meet the endpoint with 95% certainty. This translates to 60 consecutive products meeting the endpoint with a zero failure rate.[49] For other parameters that do not have an established industry practice or a definite endpoint, the FDA may request a statistical plan based on the variability of the assay before the initiation of testing. In vitro studies may be helpful in deciding whether a novel product responds in the same manner as a conventionally collected product.

Phase 2 clinical trials help to determine the kinetics of the cellular product in circulation. Both platelets and RBCs can be evaluated through these studies. These studies typically involve healthy volunteers who donate cellular products that are processed by the novel system to generate the new product. The product is then radiolabeled and reinfused into the volunteers, and serial blood samples are taken sequentially to determine the amount of the reinfused platelet product in circulation. The initial recovery and survival of the product in circulation can then be calculated from this data.

The FDA discussed standards for approval of platelet products at the July 2004 BPAC. The committee recommended (13 yes, 1 no) a recovery criteria greater than or equal to 66 percent when compared with fresh autologous platelets. The committee was less clear on its recommendations for survival greater than or equal to 66 percent (7 yes, 1 no, and 6 abstentions). Platelets manufactured with recently approved medical devices have had an autologous in vivo recovery greater than 66% and survival greater than 58% than those obtained with fresh platelets. These studies have involved 20 to 24 healthy volunteers.

As described above, for approved RBCs, the BPAC recommended that the in vivo recovery at the end of the shelf life be greater than 75%, 24 hours postinfusion of the product.[3] To assure that more than 70% of approved products would meet the criteria with 95% confidence, this would limit the number of failures in a group of 24 healthy volunteers to no more than 3.[50]

Following the phase 2 studies, manufacturers evaluate the test product in the intended population for the specific clinical application. For platelet-like products, studies have been conducted in thrombocytopenic patient population. A prospective randomized and double blinded clinical trial has been used to evaluate the prevention and reduction of bleeding in a patient population transfused either with the test product or with conventional platelets.[51] Bleeding has been evaluated with a bleeding scale similar to one developed by the World Health Organization.[52] In addition to efficacy endpoints, the trials have been also closely monitored for any adverse events. A new platelet product that is found to have significantly reduced recovery and survival would not be useful in prophylaxis of bleeding in thrombocytopenic patients but may be more suitable as therapy in an actively bleeding patient and could thus be evaluated in a specific actively bleeding patient population in comparison to conventional platelets.

Phase 3 studies for evaluation of RBCs have been performed in acutely or chronically anemic patient populations. The new product has been compared to a conventional RBC product with the endpoint being related to clinical outcomes such as recovery after surgery, length of hospital stay, and mortality for acutely anemic patients, and transfusion frequency, functional patient performance, and morbidity in chronically anemic patient population. Specific designs of clinical studies have been based on the types of transfusion products and the intended use and patient population.

Evaluations of Future Cellular Transfusion Products

New technologies and novel biologic products have the potential to transform transfusion medicine, while presenting regulatory challenges to the FDA. Recently, the FDA has created a research program called the Critical Path Initiative (CPI). Its role is to enhance the FDA's ability to evaluate product safety, efficacy, and consistency in manufacturing for new medical products.[53–55] The CPI will use cutting-edge scientific methods such as genomics and proteomics to encourage the development of new products and assess product quality and safety. The FDA's commitment is to work with manufacturers to enable the entry of safe and effective novel products to the marketplace for improvement of public health.

REFERENCES

1. US Department of Health and Human Services. The 2007 nationwide blood collection and utilization survey report. Washington, DC: DHHS; 2007. Available at: http://www.hhs.gov/ophs/bloodsafety/index.html. Accessed March 17, 2010.

2. Mollison PL, Engelfreit CP, Contreras M. Mollison's blood transfusion in clinical medicine. In: Klein HG, Anstee DJ, editors. Drug discovery today technologies. 11th edition. Massachusetts: Blackwell Publishing; 2005. p. 365–6.
3. 91st Blood Products Advisory Committee meeting. Available at: http://www.fda. gov/ohrms/dockets/ac/cber08.html. Accessed March 17, 2010.
4. Tinmouth A, Chin-Yee I. The clinical consequences of the red cell storage lesion. Transfus Med Rev 2001;15:91–107.
5. Koch CG, Li L, Sessler DI, et al. Duration of red-cell storage and complications after cardiac surgery. N Engl J Med 2008;358:1229–39.
6. Weinberg JA, McGwin G Jr, Marques MB, et al. Transfusions in the less severely injured: does age of transfused blood affect outcomes? J Trauma 2008;65:794–8.
7. Rawn J. The silent risks of blood transfusion. Curr Opin Anaesthesiol 2008;21: 664–8.
8. Fergusson D, Hutton B, Hogan DL, et al. The age of red blood cells in premature infants (ARIPI) randomized controlled trial: study design. Transfus Med Rev 2009; 23:55–61.
9. Steiner ME, Stowell C. Does red blood cell storage affect clinical outcome? When in doubt, do the experiment. Transfusion 2009;49:1286–90.
10. Roback JD, Combs MR, Grossman BJ, et al, editors. AABB technical manual. 16th edition. Bethesda (MD): AABB; 2008. p. 200–1, 285.
11. AABB American Red Cross America's Blood Centers, The Armed Services Blood Program. Circular of information for the use of human blood and blood components. Bethesda (MD): AABB; 2009. Available at: http://www.fda.gov/ BiologicsBloodVaccines/GuidanceComplianceRegulatoryInformation/Guidances/ default.htm. Accessed March 17, 2010.
12. Yoshida T, AuBuchon JP, Tryzelaar L, et al. Extended storage of red blood cells under anaerobic conditions. Vox Sang 2007;92:22–31.
13. Yoshida T, AuBuchon JP, Dumont LJ, et al. The effects of additive solution pH and metabolic rejuvenation on anaerobic storage of red cells. Transfusion 2008;48: 2096–105.
14. Dumont LJ, Yoshida T, AuBuchon JP. Anaerobic storage of red blood cells in a novel additive solution improves in vivo recovery. Transfusion 2009;49:458–64.
15. Olivier EN, Qiu C, Velho M, et al. Large-scale production of embryonic red blood cells from human embryonic stem cells. Exp Hematol 2006;34:1635–42.
16. Lu SJ, Feng Q, Park JS, et al. Biological properties and enucleation of red blood cells from human embryonic stem cells. Blood 2008;112:4475–84.
17. Douay L, Lapillonne H, Turhan AG. Stem cells—a source of adult red blood cells for transfusion purposes: present and future. Crit Care Clin 2009;25:383–98.
18. Olsson ML, Clausen H. Modifying the red cell surface: towards an ABO-universal blood supply. Br J Haematol 2008;140:3–12.
19. Bihl F, Castelli D, Marincola F, et al. Transfusion-transmitted infections. J Transl Med 2007;5:25.
20. Benjamin RJ, McCullough J, Mintz PD, et al. Therapeutic efficacy and safety of red blood cells treated with a chemical process (S-303) for pathogen inactivation: a phase III clinical trial in cardiac surgery patients. Transfusion 2005;45:1739–49.
21. Rios JA, Hambleton J, Viele M, et al. Viability of red cells prepared with S-303 pathogen inactivation treatment. Transfusion 2006;46:1778–86.
22. Solheim BG. Pathogen reduction of blood components. Transfus Apher Sci 2008; 39:75–82.
23. Cancelas JA, Dumont L, Herschel L, et al. A randomized, controlled, 2-period crossover study of recovery and lifespan of radiolabeled autologous

35-day-old red blood cells prepared with a modified S-303 treatment for pathogen inactivation. Vox Sang 2008;95(S1):8, 9.

24. Allain JP, Bianco C, Blajchman MA, et al. Protecting the blood supply from emerging pathogens: the role of pathogen inactivation. Transfus Med Rev 2005;19:110–26.

25. Jennings LK. Mechanisms of platelet activation: need for new strategies to protect against platelet-mediated atherothrombosis. Thromb Haemost 2009; 102:248–57.

26. Gaydos LA, Freireich EJ, Mantel N. The quantitative relation between platelet count and hemorrhage in patients with acute leukemia. N Engl J Med 1962; 266:905–9.

27. Truilzi DJ. Transfusion-related acute lung injury: current concepts for the clinician. Anesth Analg 2009;108:770–6.

28. Vamvakas EC. Relative safety of pooled whole blood-derived versus single-donor (apheresis) platelets in the United States: a systemic review of disparate risks. Transfusion 2009;49:2743–58.

29. Dumont LJ, Kleinman S, Murphy JR, et al. Screening of single-donor apheresis platelets for bacterial contamination: the PASSPORT study results. Transfusion 2009. [Epub ahead of print].

30. Murphy WG, Foley M, Doherty C, et al. Screening platelet concentrates for bacterial contamination: low numbers of bacteria and slow growth in contaminated units mandate an alternative approach to product safety. Vox Sang 2008;95:13–9.

31. Eder AF, Kennedy JM, Dy BA, et al. Limiting and detecting bacterial contamination of apheresis platelets: inlet-line diversion and increased culture volume improve component safety. Transfusion 2009;49:1554–63.

32. Vostal J, Mondoro T. Liquid cold storage of platelets: a revitalized possible alternative for limiting bacterial contamination of platelet products. Transfus Med Rev 1997;11:286–95.

33. Rumjantseva V, Grewal PK, Wandall HH, et al. Dual roles for hepatic lectin receptors in the clearance of chilled platelets. Nat Med 2009;15:1273–80.

34. Solheim BG, Flesland O, Seghatchian J, et al. Clinical implications of red blood cell and platelet storage lesions: an overview. Transfus Apher Sci 2004;31:185–9.

35. Lin L, Dikeman R, Molini B, et al. Photochemical treatment of platelet concentrates with amotosalen and long-wavelength ultraviolet light inactivates a broad spectrum of pathogenic bacteria. Transfusion 2004;44:1496–504.

36. Ruane PH, Edrich R, Gampp D, et al. Photochemical inactivation of selected viruses and bacteria in platelet concentrates using riboflavin and light. Transfusion 2004;44:877–85.

37. van Marwijk Kooy M, Akkerman JW, van Asbeck S, et al. UVB radiation exposes fibrinogen binding sites on platelets by activating protein kinase C via reactive oxygen species. Br J Haematol 1993;83:253–8.

38. 96th Blood Products Advisory Committee Meeting, November 2009. Available at: http://www.fda.gov/AdvisoryCommitteeMeetingMaterials/BloodVaccinesandOther Biologics/default.htm. Accessed March 17, 2010.

39. Klein HG, Glynn SA, Ness PM, et al. Research opportunities for pathogen reduction/inactivation of blood components: summary of an NHLBI workshop. Transfusion 2009;49:1262–8.

40. Bode AP, Fischer TH. Lyophilized platelets: fifty years in the making. Artif Cells Blood Substit Immobil Biotechnol 2007;35:125–33.

41. Graham SS, Gonchoroff NJ, Miller JL. Infusible platelet membranes retain partial functionality of the platelet GPIb/IX/V receptor complex. Am J Clin Pathol 2001; 115:144–7.

42. Coller BS, Springer KT, Beer JH, et al. Thromboerythrocytes. In vitro studies of a potential autologous, semi-artificial alternative to platelet transfusions. J Clin Invest 1992;89:546–55.

43. Levi M, Friederich PW, Middleton S, et al. Fibrinogen-coated albumin microcapsules reduce bleeding in severely thrombocytopenic rabbits. Nat Med 1999;5: 107–11.

44. Olsen AL, Stachura DL, Weiss MJ. Designer blood: creating hematopoietic lineages from embryonic stem cells. Blood 2006;107:1265–75.

45. Takayama N, Nishikii H, Usui J, et al. Generation of functional platelets from human embryonic stem cells in vitro via ES-sacs, VEGF-promoted structures that concentrate hematopoietic progenitors. Blood 2008;111:5298–306.

46. Vostal JG. Efficacy evaluation of current and future platelet transfusion products. J Trauma 2006;60:S78–82.

47. Draft guidance for industry for platelet testing and evaluation of platelet substitute products. 1999. Available at: http://www.fda.gov/cber/guidelines.htm. Accessed March 17, 2010.

48. Code of Federal Regulations, 21 C.F.R, Section 640.24. Washington, DC; U.S. Government Printing Office. Available at: http://www.bookstore.gpo.gov. Accessed February 12, 2010.

49. Draft guidance for industry: pre-storage leukocyte reduction of whole blood and blood components intended for transfusion. 2001. Available at: http://www.fda.gov/cber/guidelines.htm. Accessed March 17, 2010.

50. 80th Blood Products Advisory Committee Meeting, July 2004. Available at: http://www.fda.gov/ohrms/dockets/ac/cber04.html. Accessed March 17, 2010.

51. McCullough J, Vesole DH, Benjamin RJ, et al. Therapeutic efficacy and safety of platelets treated with a photochemical process for pathogen inactivation: the SPRINT trial. Blood 2004;104:1534–41.

52. Heddle NM, Cook RJ, Tinmouth A, et al. A randomized controlled trial comparing standard- and low-dose strategies for transfusion of platelets (SToP) to patients with thrombocytopenia. Blood 2009;113:1564–73.

53. Atreya CD, Epstein JS. Blood safety: opportunities and challenges addressed through critical path research at FDA. In: Lam K, Timmerman H, editors. Drug discovery today technologies. London (UK): Elsevier Ltd; 2007. p. 51–4.

54. FDA critical path initiative. Available at: http://www.fda.gov/ScienceResearch/SpecialTopics/CriticalPathInitiative/default.htm. Accessed March 17, 2010.

55. Woodcock J, Woosley R. The FDA critical path initiative and its influence on new drug development. Annu Rev Med 2008;59:1–12.

The Future of Blood Management

Jonathan H. Waters, MD

KEYWORDS
- Autotransfusion • Cell salvage • Erythrocytes
- Allogeneic transfusion • Blood management
- Point of care testing

An evolving understanding of the consequences of allogeneic blood transfusion and escalating costs of providing allogeneic blood have resulted in an interest in blood management. Understanding the consequences of allogeneic transfusion includes a recognition of the immunosuppressive effects of allogeneic transfusion,[1] a growing awareness of transfusion-related acute lung injury,[2] and a rediscovery of transfusion-associated circulatory overload.[3] More recently, interest has focused on the effect of stored blood on patient outcome.[4] Although the reports of worsened patient outcome from stored blood administration result from retrospective, observational data, animal models suggest that the goal of enhancing oxygen delivery through transfusion may not actually be improving tissue oxygen levels. In these models, functional capillary density and tissue oxygenation decrease after the transfusion of stored blood.[5,6]

Questions about clinical outcome after allogeneic transfusion are paralleled by significant economic forces, causing hospitals to evaluate their use of blood. An increasing demand for allogeneic blood has forced the donor community to become creative in finding ways of increasing the supply. Fortunately, the supply has matched the increasing demand (**Fig. 1**). Most recently, an effort has been made to reduce the minimum age for donation from 17 years of age to 16, specifically to increase the size of the donor pool.[7] Rising costs of blood products have made many hospital administrators take note of the impact that allogeneic blood has on their balance sheet. In the United States, a 17% overall increase in the cost of blood occurred between 2004 and 2006 (**Table 1**).[8] These cost increases have sizably outstripped the inflation rate over the past decade. With the cost of health care receiving unprecedented attention, this kind of cost increase will certainly attract greater scrutiny.

The initial impetus for considering transfusion alternatives was the need to care for Jehovah's Witnesses, who refuse transfusion of allogeneic blood. However, these patients use every other facet of the health care system. The question arose as to how to manage these patients when they needed procedures that classically required

Department of Anesthesiology, Magee Womens Hospital of University of Pittsburgh Medical Center, 300 Halket Street, Suite 3510, Pittsburgh, PA 15213, USA
E-mail address: watejh@upmc.edu

Clin Lab Med 30 (2010) 453–465
doi:10.1016/j.cll.2010.02.011
0272-2712/10/$ – see front matter © 2010 Elsevier Inc. All rights reserved.

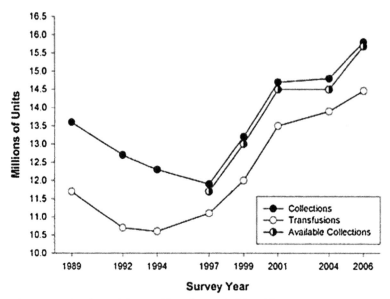

Fig. 1. Changes in supply and demand for allogeneic blood from 1989 to 2006. (*Reprinted from* The 2007 National blood collection and utilization survey report. Washington, DC: Department of Health and Human Services; 2008. p. 58; with permission.)

blood, including cardiopulmonary bypass, organ transplantation, and dialysis. To respond to this need, the "Bloodless Center" arose. Although many hospitals use this center as a marketing ploy, several facilities have become very adept at providing surgical care without the use of allogeneic transfusion. In doing so, it was discovered that the outcome for the patients treated in a bloodless fashion was comparable and sometimes better than that of the mainstream patient. For instance, one of these facilities, Englewood Hospital in New Jersey, had the lowest mortality rate for cardiac surgery in the state of New Jersey in 2006 despite using little to no allogeneic blood.[9]

BLOOD CONSERVATION STRATEGIES

Because of the issues associated with providing allogeneic blood, many experts have looked toward transfusion alternatives or blood management. The Society for the

Table 1			
Cost of blood increases from 2004 to 2006			
Product	Cost in 2006	Cost in 2004	% Change
Red blood cells	$3,427,960.62	$3,019,870.33	13%
Plasma	$239,958.40	$230,169.81	4%
Platelets	$875,189.00	$628,741.25	39%
Cryoprecipitate	$52,936.83	$47,445.90	12%
Total	$4,596,044.85	$3,926,227.29	17%

Data from The United States Department of Health and Human Services. The 2007 National Blood Collection and Utilization Survey Report. Available at: http://www.hhs.gov/ophs/bloodsafety/2007nbcus_survey.pdf. Accessed March 11, 2010.

Advancement of Blood Management defines blood management as "the appropriate provision and use of blood, its components and derivatives, and strategies to reduce or avoid the need for a blood transfusion (http://www.sabm.org/about/mission.php)." In other words, use of allogeneic blood should be confined to circumstances in which prevailing evidence suggests that patients have better clinical outcomes. Currently, this evidence is unclear, and allogeneic transfusion is administered based on historical practice and opinion.

Regarding strategies that reduce or avoid the need for transfusion, several opportunities are outlined in **Box 1**. For surgical patients, these strategies can be divided into the preoperative, intraoperative, and postoperative period. The primary strategies worth discussing in further detail involve preoperative anemia optimization, acute normovolemic hemodilution, the application of intra- and postoperative blood salvage systems, and point of care testing.

The leading risk factor for administration of allogeneic blood is the presence of anemic before the start of surgery. In many circumstances, such as trauma surgery, little can be done to change the presence of this anemia; however, in some circumstances, adequate time exists to address preoperative anemia. The environment that best presents an opportunity is orthopedic surgery, which would include joint replacement and major spine surgery. Typically, these surgeries are scheduled weeks in advance of the actual surgical time, allowing ample time for management of preexisting anemia.

To identify a preoperative anemia, the routine customs associated with scheduling a patient for surgery must be altered. The current standard is for patients to be scheduled for surgery in association with having to obtain required blood work, which is typically required by the anesthesia care team. In the current paradigm, this blood work is not reviewed until the day of surgery, leaving little opportunity to address any anemia other than through allogeneic transfusion. To best impact this process, a hemoglobin measurement must be made within the surgeons office and can occur using any number of point of care devices, with the Hemocue device being the easiest to use. Frequently, resistance to adopting this technology can be anticipated from the surgeon office staff because of the necessary licensing, training, and quality assessment needed to appropriately use these devices. Massimo Inc, a manufacturer of pulse oximetry equipment, now offers a recent technological advance in this equipment. Through the use of multiple light waves, they incorporated a continuous hemoglobin measurement device that does not fall within the rules imposed on laboratories. Although the device has not been studied extensively, it offers great promise in identifying presurgical anemia.

Once anemia is identified, the next issue is how it should be managed. Surgeons often prefer to refer the patient back to their primary care physician (PCP). The advantage here is that the PCP is typically who referred the patient to the surgeon's office. Some facilities have established internal medicine preoperative testing centers where the anemia can be managed within the hospital or clinic.

Historically, management of preoperative anemia involved aggressive use of erythropoiesis stimulating agents (ESAs) without much regard for the mechanism of the anemia. In conjunction with an increasing awareness of thrombotic complications associated with ESAs and an FDA-imposed black box warning, many practitioners have concluded that a better course of management may be to determine and address the cause of the anemia.[10] The cause can differ depending on the patient population. For a 40-year-old presenting for a hysterectomy because of dysfunctional uterine bleeding, the cause is generally obvious and related to iron deficiency from continuous blood loss. For a 70-year-old presenting for a hip replacement, the

Box 1
Components of a perioperative blood conservation program

Blood conservation should be addressed over the entire perioperative course. Components for each stage of the perioperative period are listed below:

Preoperative period

    Erythropoietin

    Androgens

    Iron, folate, B_{12} supplements

    Avoidance of anticoagulant drugs

        Nonsteroidal anti-inflammatory drugs

        Herbal supplements

        Antiplatelet drugs

        Heparin/warfarin

Intraoperative period

    Red blood cell avoidance

        Normovolemic hemodilution

        Preoperative autologous donation

        Cell salvage

Coagulation system avoidance

    Component sequestration

    Normovolemic hemodilution

Adjuncts

    Point of care testing

    Microsampling

    Drug therapy

        • Desmopressin

        • Aprotinin

        • ε-Aminocaproic acid

        • Recombinant factor VIIa

    Deliberate hypotension

    Maintenance of normothermia

    Avoidance of normal saline

    Appropriate positioning

Postoperative period

    Washed or unwashed cell salvage

    Erythropoietin/Iron

    Hyperbaric oxygen therapy

    Minimize phlebotomy

    Preoperative Anemia Optimization

differential becomes a little more difficult in that the anemia can be anemia from chronic disease or the patient might have an occult colon carcinoma. In the latter case, the patient would be far better served by having the colon carcinoma addressed before the hip replacement. As the ESAs have lost favor, intravenous iron, by itself, has been noted to frequently improve anemia of chronic disease.

Acute Normovolemic Hemodilution

Acute normovolemic hemodilution (ANH) is a technique used to reduce blood loss through temporarily storing a portion of the patient's blood volume in donor bags at the beginning of a surgical procedure. As blood is removed, blood volume is replaced using asanguinous colloid or crystalloid solutions.[11,12] This technique maintains the normal circulating blood volume, and oxygen delivery is maintained through decreases in blood viscosity. At the end of the surgical procedure, the stored blood is returned to the patient.

The goal of this technique is to create a relative anemia in the patient so that blood shed during the operative procedure effectively has a reduced number of red cells. Some simple mathematics illustrate how this technique works. A patient with a hematocrit of 40% who experiences 1000 mL of blood loss will lose 400 mL of red cells. If hemodilution has been implemented, then blood will be lost at a lower concentration. For instance, if hemodilution has resulted in a hematocrit of 25%, the same 1000 mL of blood loss will result in 250 mL of red cells lost. Thus, 150 mL of red cells have been protected from loss and can be returned to the patient at the end of surgery.

During the hemodilution process, two primary physiologic mechanisms compensate for the decrease in circulating red blood cells: cardiac output increases from increases in heart rate[13] and contractility,[14] and blood viscosity is reduced. This lowered viscosity decreases the resistance to flow so the pressure necessary to drive blood into the circulation is reduced. This lowered viscosity also improves venous return to the heart.[15] Therefore, hemodilution results in several cardiovasculature adaptations that maintain oxygen delivery.

In addition to providing a source of fresh, red blood cells, ANH will provide a source of plasma and platelets. If adequate amounts of whole blood are withdrawn (typically a liter in adults), adequate amounts of plasma and platelets are provided to correct a coagulopathy that may develop during major blood loss surgery.

Although simple in concept, ANH is often difficult to perform. If adequate blood flow into the donor bag is not maintained, then blood can clot, causing loss of valuable blood. Large-bore (9 French or larger) central venous access provides the best flow rates, although it is not always available. An acceptable alternative is to use an arterial line. Using peripheral venous access through a brachial or cephalic vein can work but not consistently, especially in small, frail elderly patients who have small peripheral veins.

The amount of blood removed for this technique is a source of controversy. If too little blood is removed, the technique lacks efficacy. If too much blood is removed, it puts the patient at risk for coronary and cerebral ischemia. Most providers will aim for a posthemodilution hemoglobin ranging from 18% to 25%. Thus, the blood available for removal depends on the starting hemoglobin.

When using ANH, the patient's preoperative hemoglobin must be optimized because anemia can be a significant obstacle to successful use of this technique. A small blood volume can also significantly limit the success of this technique. In these situations, the whole blood that is removed can be fractionated into individual components.

Fractionation can be accomplished using a blood recovery or cell salvage machine. Through changing centrifuge speeds on a standard blood salvage machine, high and low centrifugal forces separate the principal blood components. This processing is the same as the processing the blood bank uses to fractionate whole blood. Packed red cells, plasma, and platelets are individually generated during each cycle, and desired components are sequestered and held until needed. With component sequestration, varying amounts of red cells and plasma may be withheld or immediately reinfused. The generation of components instead of whole blood helps address specific patient needs without sacrificing other components. This strategy requires a much greater level of sophistication than routine ANH, and therefore is rarely used.

Blood Salvage

Blood salvage involves the collection of blood shed from a surgical site and its return to the same individual. This blood can either be washed, typically with normal saline, or can be reinfused unwashed. Washed blood salvage is typically performed in the operating room; whereas most unwashed blood salvage occurs in the postoperative environment.

Washed blood salvage

Using mathematical modeling, blood salvage seems to offer the greatest ability to help avoid allogeneic blood transfusion.[16] In some cases, little to no blood is collected and returned, but in other cases, multiple units can be salvaged and returned to a patient. **Fig. 2** shows the numbers of units produced from a cohort of 2328 patients who underwent blood salvage. Data presented on this graph were truncated at 14 units, but provide a sense of the opportunity for blood return that this technique provides.

Several aspects of blood salvage make it ideal for surgery association with major blood loss. First, major blood loss is difficult to predict accurately. Although some procedures, such as an open thoracoabdominal aneurysm repair, can guarantee sizeable blood loss, other procedures, such as open radical prostatectomy, can vary depending on patient anatomy and the skill of the surgeon. For unpredictable cases, the salvage equipment can be implemented in stages. Initially, a simple collection reservoir, a suction line, and an anticoagulant can be used. If enough blood loss occurs, the expensive components of the system can be used and blood processed.

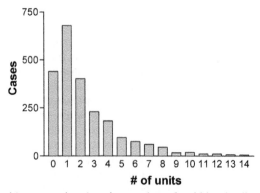

Fig. 2. A frequency histogram showing the number of red blood cell units produced from cell salvage per surgical procedure. Data were collected from 2328 patients who underwent blood salvage. Each salvaged unit was equated to an allogeneic red cell unit by measuring the hematocrit and volume of each unit, with the assumption that an allogeneic unit was approximately 200 mL of red cell volume. (*Reprinted from* Waters JR, Meier HH, Waters JH. An economic analysis of costs associated with development of a cell salvage program. Anesth Analg 2007;104:870; with permission.)

If low quantities of blood are shed, then the collection reservoir is simply discarded. In addition to this ability to stage the cost, cell salvage requires no preoperative preparation, making it ideal for unexpected major hemorrhage, such as is seen in trauma or obstetric hemorrhage.

To make washed blood salvage most effective, blood collection must be optimal. Optimization occurs using several simple concepts. First, surgical sponges must be collected and rinsed of the blood contained within them. Fully soaked gauze pads, lap sponges, or swabs may contain up to 100 mL of blood,[17] of which approximately 75% is retrievable by rinsing the sponge in a basin of isotonic solution (eg, normal saline, Ringer's Lactate, Hartmann's solution) and wrung out before discard. The rinse solution is then periodically sucked into the collection reservoir when the rinse solution seems to be grossly bloody. This practice has been reported to increase red cell retrieval rates by 28%.[18]

The second important optimization step involves ensuring that adequate anticoagulant is used while suctioning the blood. Clotting of blood in the collection system causes loss of otherwise recoverable blood and the need for reservoir and bowl replacement when large clots obstruct blood flow through the system. Either citrate or heparin can be used for anticoagulation during cell salvage. Some controversy exists as to which anticoagulant is best.[19,20]

The last step for maximizing the efficiency of blood salvage is to minimize the suction pressures applied to the blood. Normal wall suction provides −300 mmHg suction pressure. This level of suction will expose the shed blood to sizeable mechanical shear stress. Therefore, down-regulation to a level of −80 mmHg to −120 mmHg should be attempted.

Some blood salvage devices incorporate their own suction source, allowing various suction pressures to be applied. Some manufacturers require routine wall suction sources to be used. In this case, down-regulation can be implemented through adding a suction regulator. In no circumstance should down-regulation of suction pressure be implemented at the sacrifice of the surgeon being able to operate within a clear operative field.

Indications
Blood recovery may be indicated in many types of surgery, and these cases should be individualized based on the judgment of the institution and the surgeon performing the procedure. A patient's starting hematocrit, gender, age, and body weight can all influence risk associated with receiving blood components.

Contraindications
The list of contraindications to cell salvage is extensive; however, most contraindications are relative rather than absolute, meaning that few data support the danger of these proposed contraindications. When a decision is made to not use cell salvage, it must be considered in light of the known risks associated with the alternative therapy, which is allogeneic blood.

Relative contraindications to cell salvage encompass a wide range of materials that, if incorporated into the salvaged blood product, could potentially injure the patient on readministration. Definite contraindications would include anything that results in red cell lysis, such as sterile water, hydrogen peroxide, and alcohol. If blood is washed with these solutions, or a hypotonic solution is aspirated into a collection reservoir, red cell hemolysis will occur. In the presence of these contaminants, lysed cells will be washed out if the blood is adequately washed, but avoiding their incorporation into the cell salvage system is ideal. If the blood is administered without adequate washing, it could result in renal insufficiency and failure, decreases in hematocrit, elevations in serum lactate dehydrogenase, increases in total serum bilirubin concentration, disseminated intravascular coagulation, and, potentially, death.[21,22]

However, many contraindications to cell salvage are not as definitive, including blood aspirated from contaminated or septic wounds, obstetrics, and malignancy. Use of cell salvage in these circumstances varies among practices, and is advocated as safe and effective by some investigators and claimed to be dangerous by others. In many circumstances, the physician in charge should make the medical decision to proceed with autotransfusion.

In all circumstances of possible contamination, increased safety in applying cell salvage may be achieved through use of a double suction setup. In this setup, one suction line is connected to the cell salvage reservoir and used to suction blood, and the other is connected to the regular wall suction and used to aspirate the contaminant.[23–25] Use of separate suction devices minimizes contamination of the salvaged blood. The smaller the overall contamination of the salvaged red blood cells, the lower the resultant concentration in the washed product. In general, cell salvage processing can remove significant amounts of these contaminants but high enough concentrations will overwhelm the system's capabilities. Thus, every effort should be made to minimize the size of the contaminate load.

Postoperative Blood Salvage

Recovery and reinfusion of blood from surgical drains is a commonly used technique to avoid transfusion of allogeneic blood. Approximately 320,000 of these devices are used annually.[26] It is predominantly used after cardiac[27] and orthopedic procedures.[28] Typically, the blood is collected, filtered, and reinfused without washing. Because of this absence of washing, significant controversy exists about the technique. First, this salvaged blood is laden with various inflammatory mediators,[29,30] fibrin split products,[31–33] complement fractions,[34–36] interleukins,[37–39] tumor necrosis factor α,[30] and fat particles,[40] which are significantly higher than circulating levels. The most commonly reported complication after readministration of this blood is febrile reaction, which is reported to occur in between 4% and 12% of patients.[41–44] No adequately powered studies have been performed to show whether reinfusion of this blood leads to more significant complications, such as thrombotic events.

A second controversy of this technique relates to the volume of red cells returned to the patient. After cardiac surgery, blood returned to the patient averages approximately 500 mL,[45–47] whereas orthopedic procedures have greater variability, with reported blood loss ranging from 166 to 750 mL.[41,44,48] Typically, this shed blood has a hemoglobin level ranging from 20% to 30%.[31,49] Therefore, even in the most optimum circumstance, little more than a single packed red blood cell equivalent is returned to the patient. Whether this small amount of volume warrants the perceived risk associated with reinfusion of this unwashed blood is a source of debate.

Improved safety and quality management can be achieved using a processing device that concentrates the red cells and washes out contaminants. This processing can occur with wither a traditional blood salvage device or a device specifically designed for washing postoperative wound drainage blood. This specialized device (OrthoPat, CardioPat) is manufactured by Haemonetics (Braintree, MA, USA). Unfortunately, no evidence shows that this device is associated with an outcome improvement warranting its cost.

Point of care testing

A last component to blood management is that of point of care or near-care testing. With point of care testing, clinicians obtain real-time information from which to make transfusion decisions. For clinicians in the midst of major blood loss, turnaround times on laboratory data of 10 minutes are not nearly fast enough when the clinical condition of patients is rapidly changing, and they will be treated empirically with blood products without any knowledge of what blood component might be needed. With point of care testing, clinical decision-making is enhanced through using devices present at the bedside. Although the cost of having these devices in every operating room and trauma bay is prohibitive, the concept of the "laboratory on wheels" can solve this issue. (**Fig. 3**) This laboratory on wheels provides methods to determine the need for plasma, platelet, and red cell transfusion.

The benefits of using point of care testing in conjunction with an algorithm for transfusion management are sizeable. Numerous studies on patients undergoing cardiac surgery showed that the numbers of units transfused was reduced, but patient outcomes improved through fewer returns to the operating room for excessive bleeding, and they had less chest tube drainage output.[50–53]

Despite the sizeable advantages associated with point of care testing, laboratories are reluctant to lose control over the quality systems, training, and validation necessary to put these systems in place. Therefore, a strong working relationship must be developed between clinicians and laboratory technicians. Clinicians typically do not understand the regulatory oversight necessary to maintain these systems. Likewise, laboratory technicians have little insight into the management of severely bleeding patients. Thus, open dialog between both groups is necessary, with a focus on what strengthens patient care and outcomes.

An important feature of these point of care devices is that they allow for microsampling. For instance, a HemoCue hemoglobin analyzer requires 0.1 mL to obtain a hemoglobin concentration. Thus, iatrogenic anemia is not created by multiple, repetitive blood draws. This is especially important in the intensive care unit (ICU) where blood work may be required every hour. With this amount of repetitive testing, it is easily seen that a unit of packed red cell equivalents can be lost in a single day from traditional laboratory testing.

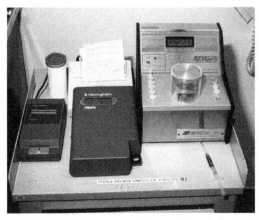

Fig. 3. The laboratory on wheels shown has a Coaguchek system for monitoring prothrombin time, partial thromboplastin time, and international normalized ratio; a Hemo-Cue device for measurement of hemoglobin concentration; and, a Sonoclot device for giving information about platelet function. Although the laboratory on wheels does not necessitate these devices, devices should be available that give information on the need for plasma, platelet, and red cell transfusion.

In conjunction with this microsampling, minimizing blood waste associated with the blood draw is important. Typically, 10 mL of blood is drawn from an arterial line before blood is drawn for laboratory sampling so that saline within the line does not dilute the blood sample. Classically, this 10 mL sample is discarded because it is considered contaminated. For certain patients in the ICU, such as those on extracorporeal membrane oxygenators, a 10-mL discard every hour can quickly result in iatrogenic anemia. To address this issue, closed blood sampling systems (VAMP system, Edwards Lifesciences, Irvine, CA, USA) allow for sampling without waste.

SUMMARY

Although this discussion is not all-inclusive, it is intended to show that many techniques can be applied to decrease the exposure to allogeneic blood. Several of these techniques require the involvement of the laboratory. Most importantly, understanding of quality systems, validation, and adequate training are characteristics unique to the laboratory environment. Other medical specialties are not as invested in standardization of processes. Because much of blood management moves traditional laboratory processes out of the laboratory and into the clinical environment, this laboratory expertise must be part of the discussion when implementing blood management programs.

REFERENCES

1. Brand A. Immunological aspects of blood transfusions. Transpl Immunol 2002;10: 183–90.
2. Kleinman S, Caulfield T, Chan P, et al. Toward an understanding of transfusion-related acute lung injury: statement of a consensus panel. Transfusion 2004;44: 1774–89.
3. Popovsky MA. Transfusion-associated circulatory overload: the plot thickens. Transfusion 2009;49:2–4.
4. Koch CG, Li L, Sessler DI, et al. Duration of red-cell storage and complications after cardiac surgery. N Engl J Med 2008;358:1229–39.
5. van Bommel J, de Korte D, Lind A, et al. The effect of the transfusion of stored RBCs on intestinal microvascular oxygenation in the rat. Transfusion 2001;41: 1515–23.
6. Tsai AG, Cabrales P, Intaglietta M. Microvascular perfusion upon exchange transfusion with stored red blood cells in normovolemic anemic conditions. Transfusion 2004;44:1626–34.
7. Shaz BH, Demmons DG, Hillyer CD. Critical evaluation of informed consent forms for adult and minor aged whole blood donation used by United States blood centers. Transfusion 2009;49:1136–45.
8. The United States Department of Health and Human Services. The 2007 National Blood Collection and Utilization Survey Report. Available at: http://www.hhs.gov/ophs/bloodsafety/2007nbcus_survey.pdf. Accessed March 11, 2010.
9. Cardiac surgery in New Jersey, 2006. Health care quality assessment. Office of the Commissioner. Available at: http://www.nj.gov/health/healthcarequality/documents/cardconsumer06.pdf. Accessed March 22, 2010.
10. Goodnough LT, Shander A, Spivak JL, et al. Detection, evaluation, and management of anemia in the elective surgical patient. Anesth Analg 2005;101:1858–61.
11. Ereth M, Oliver W, Santrach P. Perioperative interventions to decrease transfusion of allogeneic blood products. Mayo Clin Proc 1994;69:575–86.

12. Olsfanger D, Fredman B, Goldstein B, et al. Acute normovolemic hemodilution decreases postoperative allogeneic blood transfusion after total knee replacement. Br J Anaesth 1997;79:317–21.
13. Weiskopf RB, Feiner J, Hopf H, et al. Heart rate increases linearly in response to acute isovolemic anemia. Transfusion 2003;43(2):235–40.
14. Habler OP, Kleen MS, Podtschaske AH, et al. The effect of acute normovolemic hemodilution (ANH) on myocardial contractility in anesthetized dogs. Anesth Analg 1996;83:451–8.
15. Monk TG. Acute Normovolemic hemodilution. Anesthesiol Clin North America 2005;23:271–81.
16. Waters JH, Shin Jung Lee J, Karafa MT. A mathematical model of cell salvage compared and combined with normovolemic hemodilution. Transfusion 2004; 44:1412–6.
17. Ronai AK, Glass JJ, Shapiro AS. Improving autologous blood harvest: Recovery of red cells from sponges and suction. Anaesth Intensive Care 1987;15:421–4.
18. Haynes SL, Bennett JR, Torella F, et al. Does washing swabs increase the efficiency of red cell recovery by cell salvage in aortic surgery? Vox Sang 2005;88:244–8.
19. Saarla E. Autotransfusion: a review. Ann Clin Res 1981;13:48–56.
20. Oller DW, Rice CL, Herman CM, et al. Heparin versus citrate anticoagulation in autotransfusion. J Surg Res 1976;20:333–40.
21. Pierce LR, Gaines A, Varricchio F, et al. Hemolysis and renal failure associated with use of sterile water for injection to dilute 25% human albumin solution. Am J Health Syst Pharm 1998;55:1057–70.
22. From the Centers for Disease Control and Prevention. Hemolysis associated with 25% human albumin diluted with sterile water—United States, 1994–1998. JAMA 1999;281:1076–7.
23. Fong J, Gurewitsch ED, Kump L, et al. Clearance of fetal products and subsequent immunoreactivity of blood salvaged at cesarean delivery. Obstet Gynecol 1999;93:968–72.
24. Potter PS, Waters JH, Burger GA, et al. Application of cell-salvage during cesarean section. Anesthesiology 1999;90:619–21.
25. Rebarber A, Lonser R, Jackson S, et al. The safety of intraoperative autologous blood collection and autotransfusion during cesarean section. Am J Obstet Gynecol 1998;179:715–20.
26. Waters JH, Dyga RM. Postoperative blood salvage: outside the controlled world of the blood bank. Transfusion 2007;47:362–5.
27. Martin J, Robitaille D, Perrault LP, et al. Reinfusion of mediastinal blood after heart surgery. Thorac Cardiovasc Surg 2000;120:499–504.
28. Ayers DC, Murray DG, Duerr DM. Blood salvage after total hip arthroplasty. J Bone Joint Surg Am 1995;77:1347–51.
29. Sinardi D, Marino A, Chillemi S, et al. Composition of the blood sampled from surgical drainage after joint arthroplasty: quality of return. Transfusion 2005;45:202–7.
30. Dalén T, Bengtsson A, Brorsson B, et al. Inflammatory mediators in autotransfusion drain blood after knee arthroplasty, with and without leucocyte reduction. Vox Sang 2003;85:31–9.
31. Blevins FT, Shaw B, Valeri CR, et al. Reinfusion of shed blood after orthopaedic procedures in children and adolescents. J Bone Joint Surg Am 1993;75:363–71.

32. Duchow J, Ames M, Hess T, et al. Activation of plasma coagulation by retransfusion of unwashed drainage blood after hip joint arthroplasty: a prospective study. J Arthroplasty 2001;16:844–9.

33. Krohn CD, Reikeras O, Bjornsen S, et al. Fibrinolytic activity and postoperative salvaged untreated blood for autologous transfusion in major orthopaedic surgery. Eur J Surg 2001;167:168–72.

34. Andersson I, Tylman M, Bengtson JP, et al. Complement split products and proinflammatory cytokines in salvaged blood after hip and knee arthroplasty. Can J Anaesth 2001;48:251–5.

35. Bengtsson A, Avall A, Hyllner M, et al. Formation of complement split products and proinflammatory cytokines by reinfusion of shed autologous blood. Toxicol Lett 1998;100-101:129–33.

36. Jensen CM, Pilegaard R, Hviid K, et al. Quality of reinfused drainage blood after total knee arthroplasty. J Arthroplasty 1999;14:312–8.

37. Handel M, Winkler J, Hornlein RF, et al. Increased interleukin-6 in collected drainage blood after total knee arthroplasty: an association with febrile reactions during retransfusion. Acta Orthop Scand 2001;72:270–2.

38. Krohn CD, Reikeras O, Aasen AO. Inflammatory cytokines and their receptors in arterial and mixed venous blood before, during and after infusion of drained untreated blood. Transfus Med 1999;9:125–30.

39. Tylman M, Bengtson JP, Avall A, et al. Release of interleukin-10 by reinfusion of salvaged blood after knee arthroplasty. Intensive Care Med 2001;27:1379–84.

40. Parker MJ, Roberts C, Hay D. Closed suction drainage for hip and knee arthroplasty. J Bone Joint Surg Am 2004;86:1146–52.

41. Clements DH, Sculco TP, Burke SW, et al. Salvage and reinfusion of postoperative sanguineous wound drainage. A preliminary report. J Bone Joint Surg Am 1992; 74:646–51.

42. Arnestad JP, Bengtsson A, Bengtson JP, et al. Release of cytokines, polymorphonuclear elastase and terminal C5b-9 complement complex by infusion of wound drainage blood. Acta Orthop Scand 1995;66:334–8.

43. Wixson RL, Kwaan HC, Spies SM, et al. Reinfusion of postoperative wound drainage in total joint arthroplasty. Red blood cell survival and coagulopathy risk. J Arthroplasty 1994;9:351–8.

44. Faris PM, Ritter MA, Keating EM, et al. Unwashed filtered shed blood collected after knee and hip arthroplasties. A source of autologous red blood cells. J Bone Joint Surg Am 1991;73:1169–78.

45. Roberts SR, Early GL, Brown B, et al. Autotransfusion of unwashed mediastinal shed blood fails to decrease banked blood requirements in patients undergoing aortocoronary bypass surgery. Am J Surg 1991;162:477–80.

46. Eng J, Kay PH, Murday AJ, et al. Postoperative autologous transfusion in cardiac surgery: a prospective, randomized study. Eur J Cardiothorac Surg 1990;4:595–600.

47. Thurer RL, Lytle BW, Cosgrove DM, et al. Autotransfusion following cardiac operations: a randomized, prospective study. Ann Thorac Surg 1979;27:500–7.

48. Ritter MA, Keating EM, Faris PM. Closed wound drainage in total hip or total knee replacement: a prospective, randomized study. J Bone Joint Surg Am 1994;76:35–8.

49. Munoz M, Garcia-Vallejo JJ, Ruiz MD, et al. Transfusion of post-operative shed blood: laboratory characteristics and clinical utility. Eur Spine J 2004;13(Suppl 1): S107–13.

50. Nuttall GA, Oliver WC, Santrach PJ, et al. Efficacy of a simple intraoperative transfusion algorithm for nonerythrocyte component utilization after cardiopulmonary bypass. Anesthesiology 2001;94:773–81 [discussion: 775A–6A].

51. Despotis GJ, Grishaber JE, Goodnough LT. The effect of an intraoperative treatment algorithm on physicians' transfusion practice in cardiac surgery. Transfusion 1994;34:290–6.
52. Avidan MS, Alcock EL, Da Fonseca J, et al. Comparison of structured use of routine laboratory tests or near-patient assessment with clinical judgment in the management of bleeding after cardiac surgery. Br J Anaesth 2004;92:178–86.
53. Shore-Lesserson L, Manspeizer HE, DePerio M, et al. Thromboelastography-guided transfusion algorithm reduces transfusions in complex cardiac surgery. Anesth Analg 1999;88:312–9.

Recent Developments and Future Directions of Alloimmunization to Transfused Blood Products

James C. Zimring, MD, PhD

KEYWORDS

• Alloimmunization • Transfusion • Rejection • Immunity

Immunization is defined as the generation of an immune response against an antigen. Whereas immunization often is discussed as an adaptive response to foreign antigens encountered as part of a microbial infection, alloimmunization in particular is the response to antigens that differ as a function of coming from a separate member of the same species. In current medical practice, alloimmunization is perhaps most closely managed in the context of solid organ transplantation. With few exceptions, solid organs will undergo rejection by the recipient immune system in the absence of pharmacologic immunosuppression. Such appears not to be the case for transfusion, however. Outside the context of RhD, the rate of alloimmunization to red blood cell (RBC) antigens is quite low (approximately 3%) even in the absence of immunosuppressive drugs.[1,2] Alloimmunization to transfused platelets is substantially higher when focusing on responses to major histocompatability complex (MHC) I molecules (approximately 20% to 40%).[3–6] However, rates of alloimmunization to platelet-specific polymorphisms (eg, human platelet antigens) are at lower levels, similar to RBC antigens.[3–6] Alloimmunization to transfused soluble proteins also has been observed in some settings, but data on exact specificities and rates are unclear.[7] Overall, this low response rate to alloantigens is in contradistinction to antibody responses to microbial infection, which approach 100% in immunocompetent individuals; indeed, it is precisely by such serology that one monitors epidemiology of infectious pathogens.

The exact reasons why immunization to transfused blood is lower than expected is unclear, but several lines of thought have evolved. First, the extent of antigenic difference between most donor and recipient antigens is quite low. Whereas an infectious

Department of Pathology and Laboratory Medicine, Center for Transfusion and Cellular Therapies, Emory University School of Medicine, Woodruff Memorial Building Suite 7107, 101 Woodruff Circle, Atlanta, GA 30322, USA
E-mail address: jzimrin@emory.edu

Clin Lab Med 30 (2010) 467–473
doi:10.1016/j.cll.2010.02.012
0272-2712/10/$ – see front matter © 2010 Elsevier Inc. All rights reserved.

microbe may introduce numerous completely foreign proteins, most blood group antigens consist of a single amino acid difference. Also, transfused RBCs or platelets may be weakly immunogenic because of the conditions under which the antigen is encountered. Research in recent years has shown that in many cases, activation of innate immune pathways is required for acquired immunity to develop. Such activation appears to occur predominantly in response to encountering chemical motifs found on microbes but not on human tissues. Pattern recognition receptors are ligated by such motifs and provide required signals to allow the full development of immunity.[8,9] If processed and stored under sterile conditions, it is not immediately obvious how a bag of blood would deliver the requisite activation of innate immunity. Finally, transfused RBCs can introduce a large quantity of antigen that persists for a substantial amount of time, both of which are variables that often are associated with weak responses or tolerant states. Each of the variables listed has a potential role in regulating the immunogenicity of transfused blood. Understanding the factors that regulate whether an individual becomes alloimmunized is of central importance to improving transfusion management. Identification of the variables that determine alloimmunization would generate both screening tests to identify high-risk patients and also lead to the rational basis of developing therapeutic interventions.

RISK FACTORS FOR HUMORAL IMMUNIZATION TO TRANSFUSED ANTIGENS: PREDICTION AND PREVENTION
Recipient Factors Hypothesized to Regulate Alloimmunization

Although a sterile bag of blood may not have the requisite microbial products to activate innate immunity upon transfusion, it does not necessarily follow that the transfusion recipient will not have ongoing activation of innate immunity from other sources. Blood seldom is transfused into healthy people, and exposure to transfused foreign antigens may occur in the context of various underlying pathophysiologies, many of which may have a component of innate immune activation. Murine models have shown that treating recipients with activators of innate immunity can substantially increase both the frequency and magnitude of alloimmunization to an antigen on transfused RBCs.[10–13] Although this suggests a rather straightforward paradigm, additional work has suggested that not all inflammation is equivalent, and different subtypes of innate immune activation may have alternate effects upon alloimmunization.[14] Early studies in people have shown a correlation between alloimmunization and having a febrile episode in temporal association with the transfusion.[15] Much additional work, however, needs to be done to determine if inflammation really is a risk factor for alloimmunization in people, and if so, the nature of the inflammation involved.

In addition to acquired inflammation, immunogenetics outside the HLA may play a substantial role. It is known that polymorphisms in transcriptional regulators of immunoregulatory cytokines can affect rates of organ transplant rejection, but little is known about their role in alloimmunization. In addition, association of polymorphisms in coding regions of immunoregulatory gene products also has been suggested to play a role in tendency toward alloimmunization.[16]

Donor and Unit Factors Hypothesized to Regulate Alloimmunization

In addition to recipient factors, it is also possible that substances contained within transfused products may lead to innate immune activation. An obvious example would be direct microbial contamination of the blood product. Clearly, this is highly unlikely for the panel of infectious pathogens for which the blood supply is screened routinely. Moreover, the deferral of symptomatically ill donors and donors with certain pathologies decreases the likelihood of donor-derived inflammatory substances. Still, a certain number of donors would be expected to transmit relatively benign viral pathogens or have altered serum cytokines, none of which may cause substantial symptoms in the transfusion recipient but may affect immunization to transfused cells. Indeed, animal models have shown that direct addition of bacterial-like DNA sequences to blood before transfusion substantially enhances alloimmunization.[12]

There are certainly potential sources of innate immune activation distinct from microbial contamination. In particular, in nations that universally screen the blood supply for infectious pathogens, blood products are rarely if ever transfused fresh, as they need be stored at least a sufficient amount of time for pathogen screening to be performed. The approval of storage conditions for RBCs is based almost exclusively on acceptable post-transfusion survival, with little attention to other biochemical changes that may occur. It recently has been shown in a mouse model that stored RBCs are substantially more immunogenic than fresh.[17] It is currently unclear if these findings are directly applicable to human RBCs, but these data raise the distinct possibility that age-related changes damage stored cells in a way that increases immunogenicity, potentially through activation of innate immunity upon transfusion. Storage of platelet products also has been shown to result in the accumulation of immunomodulatory substances in the unit. Many of such substances are secreted by leukocytes, and filter leukoreduction has decreased the levels. Platelets themselves release immune mediators, however, including CD154.[18] Thus, a number of potential mediators can accumulate in blood products, either of microbial or endogenous origins. It long has been appreciated that patients who make one antibody tend to make additional antibodies, suggesting that factors regulating alloimmunization are more specific to recipient biology than to donor units. Donor and recipient factors are not mutually exclusive, however, as recipients may be predisposed to become alloimmunized, but only if the transfused unit also has specific properties. The exact impact of such factors on the process of alloimmunization is unclear; however, the panoply of potential substances is a likely target of both future mechanistic research and assay development for product screening.

NONANTIBODY-BASED IMMUNE RESPONSES TO TRANSFUSED ALLOANTIGENS: EFFECTS UPON TRANSPLANTATION

Transfusion immunology has its roots firmly grounded in the study of antibody responses. In fact, starting with Landsteiner's serologic analysis of the ABO system, one could argue that immunohematology has focused exclusively upon antibodies. Antibody responses, however, are just one arm of the adaptive immune system. Effector adaptive immune responses also can be carried out by CD4+ or CD8+ T cells, and innate immunity can be performed by other classes such as NK cells. In some cases (eg, $\gamma\delta$ T cells), the line between innate and adaptive immunity can be somewhat blurred.

It is certainly a legitimate question as to whether nonantibody-based immunity is of any clinical relevance whatsoever to transfusion medicine. Of potential importance is the effect that transfusion has not only on the immediate state being treated (eg, anemia or thrombocytopenia), but also effects on long-term outcome of the disease being treated. Transfusion support is an integral component of the treatment of several diseases for which the only existing cure is bone marrow or organ transplantation. In addition to the potential induction of antibodies against major histocompatability antigens (ie, MHC molecules, which can be clinically significant in their own right), cellular immunization to MHC antigens long has been appreciated to decrease success rates of transplants expressing the recognized MHC. With increased HLA matching of organs or bone marrow, the relevance of MHC immunization decreases. Indeed, when using MHC-matched (HLA identical) siblings as donors, the risk of rejection across HLA barriers is essentially zero by definition. HLA identical, however, does not mean genetically identical. Although both the donor and recipient may encode the same MHC molecules, polymorphisms in other proteins persist. Minor histocompatability antigens consist of peptides containing such polymorphisms presented by the MHC molecule. Thus, even in HLA identical donor/recipient pairs, minor antigens can serve as a vector for rejection.[19]

To the extent that minor antigens are shared on transfused blood products and the transplanted organ, transfusion has the potential to induce cellular immunity in the recipient that could participate in subsequent transplant rejection. This is perhaps most likely to occur in the setting of bone marrow transplantation, as blood and bone marrow are highly related tissues. Recent animal work has shown that transfusion of units of RBCs or platelets has the potential to induce bone marrow transplant (BMT) rejection.[20,21] It additionally has been speculated that RBC antigens that also are expressed on solid organs may play a role in contributing to solid organ rejection.[22] Such problems are most likely to occur with milder immunosuppression regimens. For example, BMT for neoplasia has a chemotherapeutic conditioning regimen sufficiently intense to make rejection highly unlikely by ablating the recipient immune system. In contrast, reduced intensity conditioning, often used for BMT for nonmalignant diseases (eg, hemoglobinopathies) would allow sufficient immunity for transfusion to prime rejection. Likewise, milder pharmacologic immunosuppression in solid organ transplant may allow such transfusion-induced rejection to occur.

So a major question to be considered in the evolution of transfusion immunology is does immunization to minor antigens actually occur in people, and if so, to what extent. Observational studies have shown a trend indicating that the more transfusions a patient receives, the more likely he or she is to reject an HLA-matched BMT under reduced intensity conditioning.[23-25] Although consistent with transfusion-induced immune-mediated BMT rejection, this is also consistent with nonimmunologic causes (eg, iron overload) or a simple correlation that more severe disease leads both to the need for more transfusions and a marrow environment less supportive of transplanted stem cells. Given the animal data supporting a direct role for immunization (the recipients in these studies had demonstrable immunity and neither bone marrow disease nor chronic transfusion), the rational basis exists for testing this hypothesis in people.[20,21] But how would such a hypothesis be evaluated? Current serologic methodologies are incapable of measuring cellular immunity in transfusion recipients. Development of robust and clinically useful tests of cellular immunity against minor antigens would have to be achieved to carry out clinical studies to directly test if the observed correlation includes immunization. Such assays might include tetramer-based flow cytometric tests, but this would require matching the HLA of tetramer regents to a recipient's HLA. Alternatively, in vitro cellular stimulation assays with recipients' leukocytes and donor antigens might be performed, using proliferation, surface marker activation, or cytokine secretion as a measure of cellular immunity. One caveat is that the validity of each of the listed approaches depends upon the assumption that peripheral circulating lymphocytes reflect the content of the immune lymphatics or bone marrow.

If experimental studies in people reflect the biology observed in mice and the correlation observed in people—namely, that transfusion immunizes recipients to minor antigens resulting in cellular immunity that predisposes to transplant rejection—the next question would become how to address the problem therapeutically. It is unclear to what extent filter leukoreduction will be effective, as minor antigens theoretically can come from nonleukocyte populations through cross-presentation of antigens by recipient antigen-presenting cells. Indeed, filter leukoreduction does not prevent transfusion-induced BMT rejection in animal models.[20,21] One could match the minor antigens; however, given the complexity of matching even the known blood group antigens, the addition of even more entities may not be logistically feasible. Because the offending antigen would have to be expressed both by peripheral blood and the target transplant, however, for any given organ the number of offending minor antigens may be small. Moreover, avoiding transfusion from the individuals who subsequently donate transplanted tissues may have some efficacy. In particular, it would be rational to predict that directed donation of blood products from the donor or other family members should be avoided, as they may share polymorphisms that constitute minor antigens. If matching is not fully feasible, then tailoring conditioning regimens or immunosuppressive approaches to the extent of pretransplant immunization may be a fruitful approach. In this way, development of the previously mentioned assays could guide therapy by informing the clinicians of pre-existing immune barriers to transplantation. Indeed, such is already common practice for humoral immunity by screening potential transplant recipients for HLA antibodies. Future developments may see the application of this approach to cellular immunity as well.

SUMMARY

Research in recent years has led to the application of evolving paradigms from the field of basic immunology to the ongoing development of the understanding of clinical transfusion-induced alloimmunization. The very concept of alloimmunization may be extending beyond the traditional antibody-based response to effector functions of cellular immunity that may affect transplantations. For both antibody responses and cellular immunity, understanding the factors that regulate why some transfusion recipients, but not others, become alloimmunized would allow both the development of clinical tests to predict patients at high risk for alloimmunization and also therapies to prevent alloimmunization. There are several factors that may precipitate activation of innate immunity, either by products in the blood unit (ie, microbial contamination, biochemical degradation, or cytokine/chemokine elaboration) or activation of innate immunity in the recipient (ie, infection, inflammatory pathology, or immunogenetics). The evolution of this field likely will consist of continuing to test potential factors in animal models with relevant follow-up studies in people, leading to tests to predict alloimmunization risk and potential approaches to decreasing alloimmunization. The clinical pathologist in general, and the transfusion medicine physician in particular, may make use of such tests and approaches in future years to better manage transfusion.

REFERENCES

1. Heddle NM, Soutar RL, O'Hoski PL, et al. A prospective study to determine the frequency and clinical significance of alloimmunization post-transfusion. Br J Haematol 1995;91:1000–5.
2. Hoeltge GA, Domen RE, Rybicki LA, et al. Multiple red cell transfusions and alloimmunization. Experience with 6996 antibodies detected in a total of 159,262 patients from 1985 to 1993. Arch Pathol Lab Med 1995;119:42–5.
3. Godeau B, Fromont P, Seror T, et al. Platelet alloimmunization after multiple transfusions: a prospective study of 50 patients. Br J Haematol 1992;81:395–400.

4. Kiefel V, Konig C, Kroll H, et al. Platelet alloantibodies in transfused patients. Transfusion 2001;41:766–70.
5. Slichter SJ. Platelet refractoriness and alloimmunization. Leukemia 1998; 12(Suppl 1):S51–3.
6. Taaning E, Simonsen AC, Hjelms E, et al. Platelet alloimmunization after transfusion. A prospective study in 117 heart surgery patients. Vox Sang 1997;72: 238–41.
7. Heal JM, Cowles J, Masel D, et al. Antibodies to plasma proteins: an association with platelet transfusion refractoriness. Br J Haematol 1992;80:83–90.
8. Medzhitov R. Recognition of microorganisms and activation of the immune response. Nature 2007;449:819–26.
9. Takeda K, Kaisho T, Akira S. Toll-like receptors. Annu Rev Immunol 2003;21: 335–76.
10. Hendrickson JE, Chadwick TE, Roback JD, et al. Inflammation enhances consumption and presentation of transfused RBC antigens by dendritic cells. Blood 2007;110:2736–43.
11. Hendrickson JE, Desmarets M, Deshpande SS, et al. Recipient inflammation affects the frequency and magnitude of immunization to transfused red blood cells. Transfusion 2006;46:1526–36.
12. Yu J, Heck S, Yazdanbakhsh K. Prevention of red cell alloimmunization by CD25 regulatory T cells in mouse models. Am J Hematol 2007;82:691–6.
13. Zimring JC, Hendrickson JE. The role of inflammation in alloimmunization to antigens on transfused red blood cells. Curr Opin Hematol 2008;15:631–5.
14. Hendrickson JE, Roback JD, Hillyer CD, et al. Discrete Toll-like receptor agonists have differential effects on alloimmunization to transfused red blood cells. Transfusion 2008;48:1869–77.
15. Yazer MH, Triulzi DJ, Shaz B, et al. Does a febrile reaction to platelets predispose recipients to red blood cell alloimmunization? Transfusion 2009;49:1070–5.
16. Tatari-Calderone Z, Minniti CP, Kratovil T, et al. rs660 polymorphism in Ro52 (SSA1;TRIM21) is a marker for age-dependent tolerance induction and efficiency of alloimmunizaiton in sickle cell disease. Mol Immunol 2009;47:64–70.
17. Hendrickson JE, Hod EA, Spitalnik SL, et al. Storage of murine red blood cells enhances alloantibody responses to an erythroid-specific model antigen. Transfusion 2009;50(3):642–8.
18. Kaufman J, Spinelli SL, Schultz E, et al. Release of biologically active CD154 during collection and storage of platelet concentrates prepared for transfusion. J Thromb Haemost 2007;5:788–96.
19. Dierselhuis M, Goulmy E. The relevance of minor histocompatability antigens in solid organ transplantation. Curr Opin Organ Transplant 2009;14:419–25.
20. Desmarets M, Cadwell CM, Peterson KR, et al. Minor histocompatability antigens on transfused leukoreduced units of red blood cells induce bone marrow transplant rejection in a mouse model. Blood 2009;114:2315–22.
21. Patel SR, Cadwell CM, Medford A, et al. Transfusion of minor histocompatability antigen-mismatched platelets induces rejection of bone marrow transplants in mice. J Clin Invest 2009;119:2787–94.
22. Lerut E, Van Damme B, Noizat-Pirenne F, et al. Duffy and Kidd blood group antigens: minor histocompatability antigens involved in renal allograft rejection? Transfusion 2007;47:28–40.
23. Deeg HJ, Self S, Storb R, et al. Decreased incidence of marrow graft rejection in patients with severe aplastic anemia: changing impact of risk factors. Blood 1986;68:1363–8.

24. Champlin RE, Horowitz MM, van Bekkum DW, et al. Graft failure following bone marrow transplantation for severe aplastic anemia: risk factors and treatment results. Blood 1989;73:606–13.

25. Gluckman E, Horowitz MM, Champlin RE, et al. Bone marrow transplantation for severe aplastic anemia: influence of conditioning and graft-versus-host disease prophylaxis regimens on outcome. Blood 1992;79:269–75.

The Platelet Storage Lesion

Dana V. Devine, PhD[a,b,*], Katherine Serrano, PhD[a,b]

KEYWORDS

- Platelet transfusion • Platelet concentrates
- Platelet storage lesion

The ability to create a platelet product for transfusion purposes has existed for more than 50 years,[1] and has contributed to fundamental changes in the practice of transfusion medicine. At the same time, this product still presents one of the major challenges to the blood bank, owing not to an inability to prepare a platelet component but because of the limitations of storing platelets under standard blood bank conditions. Depending on the jurisdiction, platelets have a maximum storage time of 3 to 7 days. In countries with a 5-day storage limit, it is estimated that upwards of 30% of the platelet inventory is discarded either by the blood supplier or the hospital blood bank. With the constraints imposed by the time to complete donor testing and shipment of product, platelet products are often received by hospital blood banks with a remaining shelf life limited to hours, further challenging inventory management practices and at times contributing to platelet shortages. This platelet storage constraint represents a significant waste of resources and is a focus of significant research effort.

There are two main reasons that platelet shelf life is limited to a small number of days. The first of these is the risk for bacterial contamination. Because the standard storage conditions for platelets consist of incubation at $22^\circ C$,[2] most commonly suspended in plasma, ideal conditions are created for the growth of most bacterial species. Thus the inoculation of only a few organisms by inadequate skin preparation during donation can lead over the time of storage to the production of large numbers of bacteria, possibly with the concomitant accumulation of large amounts of bacterial toxins and biologic response modifiers. Infusion of such a platelet product can cause death in some instances.[3] The risk for bacterial contamination of platelet products can be mitigated by bacterial testing of the product or by treatment of platelets with pathogen inactivation processes.[4] Thus, there is hope that the storage limitation imposed by bacterial risk will one day be gone.

[a] Research and Development, Canadian Blood Services, 2350 Health Sciences Mall, Vancouver, BC V6T 1Z3, Canada
[b] Pathology & Laboratory Medicine, University of British Columbia Center for Blood Research, 2350 Health Sciences Mall, Vancouver, BC V6T 1Z3, Canada
* Corresponding author. Research and Development, Canadian Blood Services, 2350 Health Sciences Mall, Vancouver, BC V6T 1Z3, Canada.
E-mail address: dana.devine@blood.ca

Clin Lab Med 30 (2010) 475–487
doi:10.1016/j.cll.2010.02.002
0272-2712/10/$ – see front matter © 2010 Elsevier Inc. All rights reserved.

However, the second reason for the limitation on platelet shelf life remains. Over the storage period, platelets begin to show evidence of a loss of quality that raises concerns about the efficacy of a transfusion that would be performed with such a product. Collectively, the loss of platelet quality over storage is known as the platelet storage lesion, or the platelet storage deficit.[5] Our current understanding of the basis of the storage lesion and the significance of ongoing research in this area is the topic of this article.

PRODUCTION OF PLATELET PRODUCTS

To understand the platelet storage lesion, it is necessary to consider the ways in which platelets are isolated for the production of platelet products used for transfusion. Centrifugation remains the basic method for the isolation of platelets; what varies is the level of sophistication. The most technically complex method for isolation of platelets for transfusion is the use of apheresis technology where all steps to the production of a unit of platelet concentrate after the placement of the needle in the donor's arm are performed in an automated fashion with no manual processing steps required and a high degree of process control.[6] All other platelet products for transfusion purposes are prepared from a whole blood donation. There are two main production protocols that are named for the preparation steps used to create them: platelet-rich plasma (PRP), and buffy coat.[7,8] The differences between the two are illustrated in **Fig. 1**. Briefly, the main difference lies in the amount of force applied in the first centrifugation step. In the buffy-coat method, a higher gravitational (g) force is applied causing the platelets and leukocytes to form a tight buffy-coat layer between the red cell and plasma layers. On the other hand, the platelet-rich plasma method uses an amount of force just sufficient to pellet the red cells and leave the platelets suspended in the plasma. At the next step of production, the buffy-coat method then uses a reduced g force to pellet the residual red cells and leukocytes and leave the platelets suspended in the plasma. In the PRP method, the platelet-rich plasma layer is subjected to a high g force to pellet the platelets and to remove most of the plasma. There are variations on these processes involving the optional use of platelet additive solutions (PAS) and pre-storage pooling either before or after production of the isolated platelets.

The production processes subject the platelets to different kinds of stresses and stimuli. For example, platelets produced by either apheresis or buffy-coat production methods show little evidence of activation.[9,10] However, platelets produced by the PRP method are visibly different; they are often temporarily aggregated together into large sheets of platelets that must be allowed to rest for the aggregation to be reversed. Some of these PRP units still contain visible aggregates at the end of the storage period. The mechanical forces to which platelets are subjected during the preparation of platelet concentrates are thought to be contributory to the development of the platelet storage lesion by providing the first insult of storage.

CHARACTERIZATION OF STORED PRODUCTS

The assessment of platelet quality is normally made in the first instance using in vitro laboratory assays. Unfortunately, there is no single laboratory test than can accurately predict the efficacy of a platelet transfusion.[11] Although this is partly because of the challenges of unraveling patient factors from platelet-concentrate factors, it is also caused by the fact that we do not fully understand the mechanisms and triggers for the development of the storage lesion. Because the preparation of platelets causes a physiologic response that resembles platelet activation, some of the laboratory tests

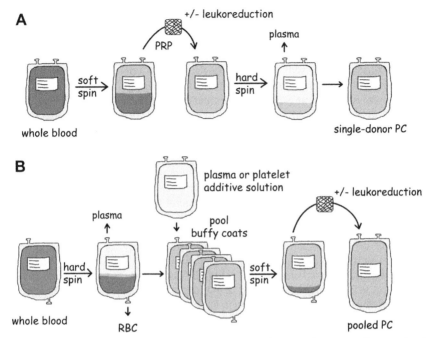

Fig. 1. PRP and buffy-coat (*top* and *bottom*) platelet production schemes. In the PRP platelet production method (*A*), whole blood is first subjected to a soft spin. The PRP is expressed off of the red blood cells and may be leukoreduced as it passes into a satellite bag. The PRP is then subjected to a hard spin and the plasma is expressed off of the sedimented platelets. The platelets are resuspended in residual plasma and stored. In the buffy-coat platelet production method (*B*), whole blood is first subjected to a hard spin. Plasma is expressed off the top and the red cells are expressed off the bottom leaving the platelet-containing buffy coat in the initial collection bag. Several buffy-coat units are pooled together with plasma or platelet additive solution and this pool is subjected to a soft spin to sediment residual red blood cells. The pooled platelet concentrate is expressed off of the red blood cells and may be leukoreduced as it passes into a final platelet-concentrate storage bag.

used to assess stored platelets are the same as those used to study platelet activation. Thus, platelet degranulation is monitored by the surface expression of CD62P or CD63, normally using flow cytometry.[12,13] Platelet degranulation may also be assessed by measuring molecules stored in platelet α-granules that are released through degranulation, such as β-thromboglobulin and platelet factor 4.[14] Platelet morphology is used as an assessment of activation state and, at the latter stages of storage, of loss of membrane integrity. A scoring system to assess stored platelets was developed 30 years ago by Kunicki and colleagues and it remains a valid tool for determining platelet quality.[15] Less widely used than CD62P and platelet morphology is the hypotonic shock response test that measures the ability of the platelet to return to its normal shape after a hypotonic challenge normally made with distilled water.[16] Light scattering is used to assess the return to discoid shape using the purpose-built SPA-2000 (ChronoLog, Havertown, PA, USA), an instrument that is similar to a platelet aggregometer. In parallel, the extent-of-shape-change test is often conducted, which measures the amount of shape change that the platelet undergoes in response to a preset dose of adenosine diphosphate (ADP).[17] Because platelets are stored at room temperature, they remain quite metabolically active compared with cells stored under refrigeration. For this reason, the assessment of platelets during storage often includes measures of the glucose and lactate concentrations. The deterioration of platelets is also associated with a loss of buffering capacity in the unit and a drop in pH may occur. A drop of platelet pH to 6.2 or below markedly reduces the in vivo survival of such platelets upon transfusion.[18] Finally, because in the early days of platelet storage the level of oxygen in the platelet storage container was found to have a significant impact on platelet quality, the pO2 and pCO2 are monitored to ensure sufficient gas exchange has occurred during storage. In most laboratories, the glucose, lactate, pH, pO2, and pCO2 measurements are readily made using a chemistry analyzer.

There are some newer platelet-specific tests being applied to the study of stored platelets. If platelets are of poor quality either because of overt activation or general deterioration, the membrane loses its ability to maintain normal lipid asymmetry and phosphatidylserine becomes expressed on the outer membrane leaflet. This characteristic can be measured using the binding of annexin V, which has a high affinity for anionic phospholipids.[19] Once again, this measurement is normally made using flow cytometry. Furthermore, a novel light-scattering technology for the assessment of platelet quality has recently been developed.[20,21]

A panel of typical measurements of a set of buffy coat-derived platelet concentrates stored for up to 9 days is shown in **Fig. 2**. Although the exact level of an analyte may differ from unit to unit or from laboratory to laboratory (especially for CD62P measurements), the trend lines of these data are quite consistent across blood products and storage containers. In these graphs, the platelet storage lesion is evidenced by an unrelenting loss of platelet functional responses and increasing evidence of some sort of platelet-activation process or at least a process that mimics platelet activation. If one makes such measurements across the three main types of platelet concentrates (apheresis, whole blood-derived by PRP, and whole blood-derived by buffy coat), one sees evidence of higher levels of platelet activation in the PRP platelets compared with the other two, however, by the end of licensable storage period of 5 to 7 days, most of this difference has disappeared.[9,10] This observation suggests that the ongoing development of the platelet storage lesion is influenced by factors occurring later than processing steps per se.

Almost all of the tests described earlier are restricted in their application to research investigations or to production facilities with more sophisticated laboratory facilities. In the routine platelet-production laboratory, the quality-control assessments made on platelet concentrates generally include only those measurements required by various standards bodies: platelet concentrate volume, platelet count, pH of the unit, and residual leukocyte count if claims of leukoreduction are made.[22] In addition, immediately before distribution to hospitals a visual inspection is made that often includes an assessment of platelet swirl, an at best semiquantitative reflection of the degree of discoid shape of the platelets within the bag.[23] Platelets with no measurable swirl have predominantly lost their discoid shape. Because rounding of platelets is consistent with loss of membrane integrity, platelets lacking swirl often show unacceptably low pH. The absence of swirling has been reported to be highly predictive of poor transfusion outcome and as a result, visible swirl is suggested to be a good first-line assessment of platelet quality.[24]

RELATIONSHIP BETWEEN IN VITRO AND IN VIVO STUDIES

The ability of stored platelets to remain in the circulation of a transfusion recipient post-transfusion can be measured using well-established in vivo viability

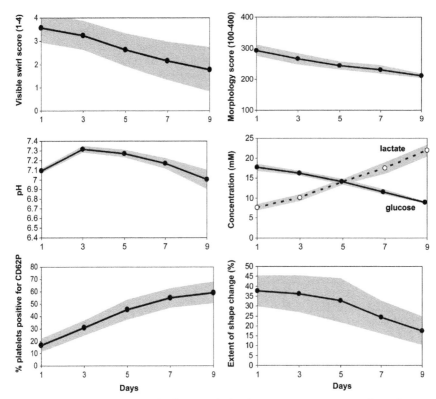

Fig. 2. Typical in vitro assay results for stored platelet concentrates up to 9 days of storage. Visible swirl and morphology scoring give an indication of the changing platelet shape. Glucose and lactate concentrations reflect the rate of platelet metabolism. CD62P expression gives an indication of platelet activation level as measured through degranulation. Extent of shape change is an indicator of platelet responsiveness to ADP. The pH decreases may reflect either loss of metabolic integrity or the presence of contaminating bacteria. The data represent the average trend for each measurement ±1 standard deviation (gray error bands).

measurements.[25] Stored platelets are radiolabelled so that they can be traced when reinfused into volunteer study subjects. The first sample withdrawn from the transfusion recipient will give an indication of the percent recovery of platelets in the circulation. Samples continue to be withdrawn at specified time intervals and from these it can be determined what the length of circulation in time of the stored platelets is, which is known as the survival. In vivo viability studies are not straightforward to perform so it would be desirable to have an in vitro assay that could predict transfusion outcome. In 2004 an international forum concluded that an in vitro platelet assay capable of predicting in vivo platelet function post-transfusion did not yet exist.[11] However, many of the forum respondents identified visible swirl, extent of shape change, hypotonic shock response, and pH as the best of the current assays based on varying degrees of correlation with in vivo viability measurements. This finding somewhat echoes the findings of a comprehensive review from 1994 that found that in vitro assessments in which a correlation with in vivo viability was seen included measures of platelet morphology, as determined with morphology scores and extent of shape change; hypotonic shock response; pH; maintenance of adenosine triphosphate (ATP) levels; and reduced lactate production. Platelet α-granule release or platelet lysis, determined through measurements of platelet factor 4, beta-thromboglobulin, or lactate dehydrogenase, did not appear to be good predictors of in vivo platelet function.[26] Some of the correlations identified between in vitro assays and in vivo viability measurements can be seen in **Table 1**.

Although morphology as determined either by visible swirl, microscopy, or with extent-of-shape-change measurement suggests promise as an indicator of in vivo viability, it is interesting to note that in studies where platelet shape change has been inhibited pharmacologically there has not been a corresponding improvement

Table 1
Correlations between some commonly conducted in vitro platelet quality measures and in vivo viability

| Measure | Correlation with Recovery | | Correlation with Survival | | References |
	r	Significant	r	Significant	
pH	—	Yes (low pH)	—	—	Murphy et al [18]
	0.88[a]	Yes	0.84[a]	Yes	Goodrich et al[27]
Visible swirl	—	Yes[b]	—	—	Bertolini et al[24]
	0.66[a]	No	0.49[a]	No	Goodrich et al[27]
Extent of shape change	0.95[c]	Yes	—	—	Murphy et al[28]
	0.51	Yes	0.49	Yes	Holme et al[29]
	0.45	Yes	—	—	Heaton et al[30]
	—	—	0.61	Yes	Moroff et al[31]
	0.40	Yes	0.50	Yes	Holme et al[32]
Hypotonic shock response	0.65	Yes	0.54	Yes	Holme et al[29]
	0.39	Yes	0.40	Yes	Holme et al[32]
Lactate production	—	—	−0.62	Yes	Heaton et al[30]
	—	—	−0.67	Yes	Moroff et al[31]
	−0.41	Yes	−0.39	Yes	Holme et al[32]
	−0.91[a]	Yes	−0.81[a]	Yes	Goodrich et al[27]
Glucose consumption	0.84[a]	No	0.78[a]	No	Goodrich et al[27]
Morphology	—	No[d]	—	No[d]	Mintz et al[44]
	0.65[a]	No	0.51[a]	No	Goodrich et al[27]
Surface CD62P	−0.55	Modest	—	—	Rinder et al[33]
	−0.58[b]	Yes	—	—	Triulzi et al[34]
	−0.28	Poor	−0.42	Modest	Holme et al[32]
	—	—	—	Yes	Dumont et al[35]
	−0.84[a]	No	−0.69[a]	No	Goodrich et al[27]
ATP	—	No	—	No	Holme et al[32]
Surface CD42b	—	Yes	—	—	Holme et al[36]
	—	No	—	No	Holme et al[32]
pO$_2$	—	—	0.63	Yes	Heaton et al[30]
	—	No	—	No	Holme et al[32]
	−0.41[a]	No	0.54[a]	No	Goodrich et al[27]
pCO$_2$	0.64[a]	No	0.59[a]	No	Goodrich et al[27]

[a] UV-treated platelets.
[b] Recovery as measured by corrected count increment (CCI 30 min or 1 h).
[c] Platelets stored on an elliptical agitator.
[d] Morphology measured with Noninvasive Assessment of Platelet Shape and Concentration (NAPSAC, Beecher Medical, Silver Spring, MD, USA) device.

in platelet survival.[37] This finding demonstrates that platelet discoid shape alone is not responsible for in vivo viability. The platelet activation marker, CD62P has shown both decent and poor correlation with in vivo viability. A possible explanation for this inconsistency is that platelet activation/degranulation is an independent process that sometimes, but not always, runs in parallel to the mechanism that leads to decreasing platelet viability. Supporting the hypothesis that CD62P expression is not related to platelet viability post-transfusion is a study that showed that autologously transfused baboon platelets that had been pre-activated with thrombin continued to circulate and function despite expressing CD62P.[38] However, CD62P is an effective measure of platelet activation and as such remains a valuable piece of information to understanding the effects of new methods of preparation and storage on platelets.

Poor correlations between in vitro platelet assays and in vivo recovery and survival measurements may not necessarily indicate a failure of the assay to reflect platelet viability considering that in vivo assays may not accurately reflect platelet viability. It has therefore been suggested that a better way to approach the issue of prediction is to determine whether conditions showing loss of in vivo viability are associated with corresponding changes of in vitro measurements.[39] A study using this approach reported that a production method resulting in higher in vivo platelet viability was associated with lower CD62P expression levels and a higher morphology score as might be expected. Unexpectedly, higher in vivo viability was also associated with lower pH and lower glucose levels.[40] In the quest for an in vitro assay that can predict in vivo outcome, one must also consider that the platelet storage lesion appears to be somewhat reversible; platelets regain lost function after transfusion.[41] This recovery appears to depend on the environment of the platelets and can be reproduced with the addition of fresh plasma or even somewhat by changes in pH.[42–44] This fact may also help to explain why poor correlations between in vitro assays and in vivo survivability are sometimes seen.

SIGNIFICANCE FOR CLINICAL TRANSFUSION OUTCOME

One of the great difficulties in assessing technological changes to platelet products is how to determine whether the product will be clinically efficacious. The gold standard testing is the use of radiolabelled platelet survival and recovery in normal volunteers.[45] However, this kind of study is not without pitfalls. In the first place, the method is expensive and can only be conducted in a laboratory with skilled platelet investigators. Furthermore, the use of radionuclides in healthy volunteers is legally prohibited in some jurisdictions thereby further limiting the ability of researchers to use this kind of gold-standard testing. For some regulatory authorities, notably the US Food and Drug Administration, the analysis of radiolabelled survival and recovery is an expectation of licensure of new technologies. Not surprisingly, this level of complexity and cost is a barrier to the introduction of new technologies. Furthermore, platelet products that are in widespread use today when assessed in these tests may prove to be inadequate when compared with other standard preparations.[40] Perhaps of equal importance is the fact that the behavior of stored platelets that are radiolabelled and reinfused into an individual with a normal platelet count may not give the same sort of information as studies in patients who are thrombocytopenic. There is little evidence that patients receiving platelets that have been stored in plasma for at least 7 days have any increased bleeding risk in comparison to patients receiving fresh platelets.[46] The existing literature is lacking studies to support the widespread clinical practice of platelet storage for up to 7 days. One of the significant challenges in assessing the significance of the platelet storage lesion on the clinical efficacy of a transfusion has been the design of the few studies that have examined this question. It is most common to study patients undergoing prophylactic platelet transfusion, usually patients under treatment for hematologic malignancies or undergoing hematopoietic progenitor cell transplantation. This is clinically a different set of circumstances than the provision of platelet products for patients who are actively bleeding, and factors that influence platelet transfusion efficacy in one setting do not necessarily transfer to the other. The transfusion of platelets to patients who are actively bleeding usually stops the bleeding unless other factors are present, and this is often independent of any increase in the post-transfusion platelet count or corrected count increment (CCI). For example, the transfusion of platelets expressing high levels of surface phosphatidylserine (as expressed by annexin V-binding) or activated integrin complexes will be primed for participation in adhesion and aggregation reactions. These platelets may actually be a better product for patients who are actively bleeding. However, that same platelet preparation may have a somewhat shortened survival time in patients who do not have active bleeding or other such confounding factors. The use of such platelet products may shorten the interval between prophylactic platelet transfusions because of decreases in circulation residency time. At least in North America, most platelet transfusions are given prophylactically, so the impact of the platelet storage lesion on the use of a country's overall platelet inventory becomes quite significant. A significant shortening of the transfusion interval in patients receiving 5- to 7-day stored platelet products translates into many more donor exposures over the course of treatment.[47] Thus, there is a need to consider specific patient factors when issuing platelets from the blood bank and the characteristics of the platelet unit itself.

BIOCHEMICAL INVESTIGATIONS OF THE STORAGE LESION

In addition to the in vitro tests described earlier that are used to assess platelet concentrate quality, other approaches have been taken to attempt to understand the platelet storage lesion. The observation that many of the ongoing changes in stored platelets are similar to changes seen after platelets are exposed to known platelet agonists have led to the focus of many of the storage-lesion studies on aspects of platelet activation, either induced by shear stress during production, by the release of compounds from passenger leukocytes or other platelets, or by the activity of molecules present in the accompanying plasma.

The natural history of platelet formation has also been proposed to play a role in the development of the platelet storage lesion. One reasonable postulated mechanism for platelet deterioration over the storage period has been the onset of apoptosis.[19] Many of the proteins that become activated are part of well-described apoptosis pathways; however, studies also find that known inhibitors of apoptosis are generally not able to block platelet storage lesion development.[48] Whether this suggests that some apoptotic processes are already activated in the megakaryocyte during proplatelet formation or that the process is simply difficult to inhibit in stored platelet concentrates is not yet known.

The obvious conclusion from the results of all of these studies has been that the development of the platelet storage lesion is a multifactorial process. Although this is highly likely, the differences between the rates of platelet storage lesion development in platelet concentrates produced by different processes suggests that the negative effects of these processes can in fact be ameliorated to some extent.

Many of the biochemical changes reported in platelets over the storage period are similar to changes seen when platelets that have not been stored or processed come in contact with harsh physical processes, such as cardiopulmonary bypass pumps, or with bioincompatible surfaces. These data suggest that it is important to consider not only improvements to the processing of components but also to the post-preparation conditions under which platelets are stored. Some research efforts are underway to modify the surface of blood bags to make a more biocompatible storage container.

Studies of the platelet storage lesion have reported an increase in the surface expression of the integrin complex GPIIb-IIIa.[49] Although this was initially interpreted as activation-induced expression of a pool of protein synthesized by the megakaryocyte, it is now apparent that platelets have an active protein synthesis that occurs throughout the storage period.[50] Furthermore, platelet proteomic studies have shown several protein changes occurring over storage that are suggestive of the renewal of a set of proteins that are involved in platelet cytoskeleton integrity or signaling pathways.[51,52] The mRNA in platelets appears to be unusually long lived compared with nucleated cells, yet not all messages are preserved. The specificity of this response begs the question as to whether this process represents some sort of cellular repair mechanism that platelets use in the absence of the full protein synthetic machinery of a nucleated cell.

As discussed earlier, there is no single laboratory test that can accurately predict the behavior of platelets when transfused. However, new scientific approaches to the platelet storage lesion may identify new targets for the development of quality control assays. Several laboratories have recently begun to apply the science of proteomics to the study of platelet storage and these findings have been recently reviewed.[53]

IMPACT OF NOVEL TECHNOLOGIES

The past decade has brought two interesting technologies into widespread use: PAS and pathogen inactivation.[54,55] Both of these have the potential to influence the development of the platelet storage lesion. The main driver for the development of solutions that could be added to platelets for storage purposes was to divert the most plasma possible to fractionation. Given the success of red cell additives in improving the quality of stored red blood cell concentrates, the concept of PAS seems to be a worthy effort to also improve the quality of stored platelets. The design of the PAS was conducted in large part with the 5-day outdate in mind, although some studies have shown good in vitro storage characteristics for storage periods approaching 2 weeks.[56] Now that there is widespread bacterial testing in place for platelets, interest has grown to determine whether platelets stored for longer periods in PAS have acceptable efficacy. It is clear that the earlier-generation PAS solutions, such as T-sol, do not preserve platelet characteristics in such a way that there is no observable difference when platelets are transfused in a 5- to 7-day window.[57] This important issue will need to be addressed going forward. Indeed, incremental improvement to PAS has produced third-generation products that show improved storage characteristics and research effort in this area continues.[58,59] As more becomes understood about the etiology of the platelet storage lesion, it should be possible to improve on the design of additive solutions to minimize their impact on the development of the storage lesion, or preferably to design them to actively inhibit its formation.

Pathogen reduction offers one of the most exciting developments in blood safety in decades. This technology involves the treatment of platelet concentrates with processes that destroy nucleic acids thereby preventing the replication of pathogenic organisms, or even the ongoing viability of passenger leukocytes. The first technologies to arrive in the marketplace involve the exposure of platelets to cross-linker chemicals that must be subsequently activated by UV light, or in one case, exposure to UV light alone.[60–62] One process requires an additional filtration step to remove the cross-linking agent. There is a clear trade-off in the application of pathogen reduction technologies between an increased margin of safety for the recipient in pathogen transmission or the negative effects of passenger leukocytes and the decrease of product efficacy. Although the randomized, controlled trials conducted to license these products showed general therapeutic equivalence, there is a clear impact of the additional processing steps on the platelet transfusion outcome in recipients.[63] It is not the additional filtration step that is responsible for loss of platelet quality induced by pathogen reduction technologies because these effects are also seen in those systems that do not require removal of a crosslinker.[64]

Other research developments will also ultimately have an impact on the evolution of the storage lesion. One interesting area is research to improve the processing and storage of components. This effort will lead to the consideration of the impact of the processing equipment and the storage container rather than the additive solution. The storage of platelets in a flexible plastic container is less than ideal for product inventory management, and the requirements for narrowly controlled storage temperature of 20 to 24°C under conditions of agitation further complicate the storage of platelet concentrates. The issues of container biocompatibility have received little attention to date, but may actually be one of the potential sources for the ongoing stimulus for storage lesion development post processing.

WHAT DOES THE FUTURE HOLD?

Most predictions of the future prove to be wildly incorrect either in substance or timelines, and any guesses as to the status of the platelet storage lesion in 2010 are likely to meet a similar fate. However, given the pace of change in transfusion medicine, it is likely that the storage lesion will still be a feature of the landscape a decade from now, although we are likely to have a better understanding of its mechanistic properties. Much work still remains to figure out how to keep platelets of the best quality possible during the storage period, especially in the face of new assaults on their integrity, such as pathogen-reduction technologies.

REFERENCES

1. Dillard JH, Brecher G, Cronkite EP. Separation, concentration, and transfusion of platelets. Proc Soc Exp Biol Med 1951;78(3):796–9.
2. Murphy S, Gardner FH. Effect of storage temperature on maintenance of platelet viability—deleterious effect of refrigerated storage. N Engl J Med 1969;280(20): 1094–8.
3. Lee J-H. Bacterial Contamination of Platelets Workshop. U.S. Department of Health and Human Services Food and Drug Administration Center for Biologics Evaluation and Research. Bethesda (MD), September 24, 1999. p. 70–83.
4. Blajchman MA, Beckers EAM, Dickmeiss E, et al. Bacterial detection of platelets: current problems and possible resolutions. Transfus Med Rev 2005;19(4):259–72.
5. Murphy S, Gardner FH. Platelet storage at 22 degrees C; metabolic, morphologic, and functional studies. J Clin Invest 1971;50(4):370–7.
6. Simon TL. The collection of platelets by apheresis procedures. Transfus Med Rev 1994;8(2):132–45.
7. Sweeney JD, Holme S, Heaton WA, et al. White cell-reduced platelet concentrates prepared by in-line filtration of platelet-rich plasma. Transfusion 1995; 35(2):131–6.

8. Murphy S. Platelets from pooled buffy coats: an update. Transfusion 2005;45(4): 634–9.
9. Vassallo RR, Murphy S. A critical comparison of platelet preparation methods. Curr Opin Hematol 2006;13(5):323–30.
10. Levin E, Culibrk B, Gyongyossy-Issa MI, et al. Implementation of buffy coat platelet component production: comparison to platelet-rich plasma platelet production. Transfusion 2008;48(11):2331–7.
11. Pietersz RN, Engelfriet CP, Reesink HW, et al. Evaluation of stored platelets. Vox Sang 2004;86(3):203–23.
12. Divers SG, Kannan K, Stewart RM, et al. Quantitation of CD62, soluble CD62, and lysosome-associated membrane proteins 1 and 2 for evaluation of the quality of stored platelet concentrates. Transfusion 1995;35(4):292–7.
13. Kannan K, Divers SG, Lurie AA, et al. Cell surface expression of lysosome-associated membrane protein-2 (lamp2) and CD63 as markers of in vivo platelet activation in malignancy. Eur J Haematol 1995;55(3):145–51.
14. Kaplan KL, Owen J. Plasma levels of β-thromboglobulin and platelet factor 4 as indices of platelet activation in vitro. Blood 1981;57(2):199–202.
15. Kunicki TJ, Tuccelli M, Becker GA, et al. A study of variables affecting the quality of platelets stored at "room temperature". Transfusion 1975;15(5):414–21.
16. Kim BK, Baldini MG. The platelet response to hypotonic shock. Its value as an indicator of platelet viability after storage. Transfusion 1974;14(2):130–8.
17. Holme S, Murphy S. Quantitative measurements of platelet shape by light transmission studies; application to storage of platelets for transfusion. J Lab Clin Med 1978;92(1):53–64.
18. Murphy S, Sayar SN, Gardner FH. Storage of platelet concentrates at 22°C. Blood 1970;35(4):549–57.
19. Li J, Xia Y, Bertino AM, et al. The mechanism of apoptosis in human platelets during storage. Transfusion 2000;40(11):1320–9.
20. Maurer-Spurej E, Labrie A, Pittendreigh C, et al. Platelet quality measured with dynamic light scattering correlates with transfusion outcome in hematologic malignancies. Transfusion 2009;49(11):2276–84.
21. Maurer-Spurej E, Brown K, Labrie A, et al. Portable dynamic light scattering instrument and method for the measurement of blood platelet suspensions. Phys Med Biol 2006;51(15):3747–58.
22. Guide to the preparation, use, and quality assurance of blood components. 13th edition. Strasbourg (France): Council of Europe Publishing; 2007.
23. Mathai J, Resmi KR, Sulochana PV, et al. Suitability of measurement of swirling as a marker of platelet shape change in concentrates stored for transfusion. Platelets 2006;17(6):393–6.
24. Bertolini F, Agazzi A, Peccatori F, et al. The absence of swirling in platelet concentrates is highly predictive of poor posttransfusion platelet count increments and increased risk of a transfusion reaction. Transfusion 2000;40(1):121–2.
25. Holme S, Heaton A, Roodt J. Concurrent label method with 111In and 51Cr allows accurate evaluation of platelet viability of stored platelet concentrates. Br J Haematol 1993;84(4):717–23.
26. Murphy S, Rebulla P, Bertolini F, et al. In vitro assessment of the quality of stored platelet concentrates. Transfus Med Rev 1994;8(1):29–36.
27. Goodrich RP, Li J, Pieters H, et al. Correlation of in vitro platelet quality measurements with in vivo platelet viability in human subjects. Vox Sang 2006;90:279–85.
28. Murphy S, Kahn RA, Holme S, et al. Improved storage of platelets for transfusion in a new container. Blood 1982;60(1):194–200.

29. Holme S, Heaton WA, Courtright M. Improved in vivo and in vitro viability of platelet concentrates stored for seven days in a platelet additive solution. Br J Haematol 1987;66(2):233–8.

30. Heaton WAL, Holme S, Keegan T. Development of a combined storage medium for 7-day storage of platelet concentrates. Br J Haematol 1990;75(3):400–7.

31. Moroff G, Holme S, George VM, et al. Effect on platelet properties of exposure to temperatures below 20°C for short periods during storage at 20 to 24°C. Transfusion 1994;34(4):317–21.

32. Holme S, Sweeney JD, Sawyer S, et al. The expression of p-selectin during collection, processing, and storage of platelet concentrates: relationship to loss of in vivo viability. Transfusion 1997;37(1):12–7.

33. Rinder HM, Murphy M, Mitchell JG, et al. Progressive platelet activation with storage: evidence for shortened survival of activated platelets after transfusion. Transfusion 1991;31(5):409–14.

34. Triulzi DJ, Kickler TS, Braine HG. Detection and significance of alpha granule membrane protein 140 expression on platelets collected by apheresis. Transfusion 1992;32(6):529–33.

35. Dumont LJ, AuBuchon JP, Whitley P, et al. Seven-day storage of single-donor platelets: recovery and survival in an autologous transfusion study. Transfusion 2002;42(7):847–54.

36. Holme S, Bode A, Heaton WA, et al. Improved maintenance of platelet in vivo viability during storage when using a synthetic medium with inhibitors. J Lab Clin Med 1992;119(2):144–50.

37. Hoffmeister KM, Felbinger TW, Falet H, et al. The clearance mechanism of chilled blood platelets. Cell 2003;112(1):87–97.

38. Michelson AD, Barnard MR, Hechtman HB, et al. In vivo tracking of platelets: circulating degranulated platelets rapidly lose surface P-selectin but continue to circulate and function. Proc Natl Acad Sci U S A 1996;93(21):11877–82.

39. Holme S. In vitro assays used in the evaluation of the quality of stored platelets: correlation with in vivo assays. Transfus Apheresis Sci 2008;39:161–5.

40. Arnold DM, Heddle NM, Kulczycky M, et al. In vivo recovery and survival of apheresis and whole blood-derived platelets: a paired comparison in healthy volunteers. Transfusion 2006;46(2):257–64.

41. Holme S. Storage and quality assessment of platelets. Vox Sang 1998; 74(Suppl 2):207–16.

42. Rinder HM, Snyder EL, Tracey JB, et al. Reversibility of severe metabolic stress in stored platelets after in vitro plasma rescue or in vivo transfusion: restoration of secretory function and maintenance of platelet survival. Transfusion 2003;43:1230–7.

43. Mondoro TH, Shafer BC, Vostal JG. Restoration of in vitro responses in platelets stored in plasma. Am J Clin Pathol 1999;111(5):693–9.

44. Mintz PD, Anderson G, Avery N, et al. Assessment of the correlation of platelet morphology with in vivo recovery and survival. Transfusion 2005;45(Suppl 2): 72S–80S.

45. Snyder EL, Moroff G, Heaton SA. Recommended methods for conducting radiolabeled platelet survival studies. Transfusion 1986;26(1):37–42.

46. Heddle NM, Arnold DM, Boye D, et al. Comparing the efficacy and safety of apheresis and whole blood-derived platelet transfusions: a systematic review. Transfusion 2008;48(7):1447–58.

47. Pereira A, Sanz C. Effect of extending the platelet storage time on platelet utilization: predictions from a mathematical model of prophylactic platelet support. Transfus Med 2007;17(2):119–27.

48. Bradley AJ, Read BL, Levin E, et al. Small-molecule complement inhibitors cannot prevent the development of the platelet storage lesion. Transfusion 2008;48(4):706–14.

49. Fijnheer R, Modderman PW, Veldman H, et al. Detection of platelet activation with monoclonal antibodies and flow cytometry. Changes during platelet storage. Transfusion 1990;30(1):20–5.

50. Thon JN, Devine DV. Translation of glycoprotein IIIa in stored blood platelets. Transfusion 2007;47(12):2260–70.

51. Thiele T, Steil L, Gebhard S, et al. Profiling of alterations in platelet proteins during storage of platelet concentrates. Transfusion 2007;47(7):1221–33.

52. Thon JN, Schubert P, Duguay M, et al. Comprehensive proteomic analysis of protein changes during platelet storage requires complementary proteomic approaches. Transfusion 2008;48(3):425–35.

53. Schubert P, Devine DV. Proteomics meets blood banking: Identification of protein targets for the improvement of platelet quality. J Proteomics 2010;73(3):436–44.

54. van der Meer PF. Platelet additive solutions: a future perspective. Transfus Clin Biol 2007;14(6):522–5.

55. Blajchman MA. Protecting the blood supply from emerging pathogens: the role of pathogen inactivation. Transfus Clin Biol 2009;16(2):70–4.

56. van der Meer PF, Pietersz RNI, Reesink HW. Storage of platelets in additive solution for up to 12 days with maintenance of good in-vitro quality. Transfusion 2004; 44(8):1204–11.

57. Diedrich B, Ringden O, Watz E, et al. A randomized study of buffy coat platelets in platelet additive solution stored 1–5 versus 6–7 days prior to prophylactic transfusion of allogeneic haematopoietic progenitor cell transplant recipients. Vox Sang 2009;97(3):254–9.

58. Diedrich B, Sandgren P, Jansson B, et al. In vitro and in vivo effects of potassium and magnesium on storage up to 7 days of apheresis platelet concentrates in platelet additive solution. Vox Sang 2008;94(2):96–102.

59. Zhang JG, Carter CJ, Culibrk B, et al. Buffy-coat platelet variables and metabolism during storage in additive solutions or plasma. Transfusion 2008;48(5): 847–56.

60. Lin L, Cook DN, Wiesehahn GP, et al. Photochemical inactivation of viruses and bacteria in platelet concentrates by use of a novel psoralen and long-wavelength ultraviolet light. Transfusion 1997;37(4):423–35.

61. Ruane PH, Edrich R, Gampp D, et al. Photochemical inactivation of selected viruses and bacteria in platelet concentrates using riboflavin and light. Transfusion 2004;44(6):877–85.

62. Mohr H, Gravemann U, Bayer A, et al. Sterilization of platelet concentrates at production scale by irradiation with short-wave ultraviolet light. Transfusion 2009;49(9):1956–63.

63. McCullough J, Vesole DH, Benjamin RJ, et al. Therapeutic efficacy and safety of platelets treated with a photochemical process for pathogen inactivation: the SPRINT Trial. Blood 2004;104(5):1534–41.

64. AuBuchon JP, Herschel L, Roger L, et al. Efficacy of apheresis platelets treated with riboflavin and ultraviolet light for pathogen reduction. Transfusion 2005; 45(8):1335–41.

Governance in the European Union: The European Blood Directive as an Evolving Practice

Hannes Hansen-Magnusson, MA

KEYWORDS

- European Blood Directive • Blood donation
- Blood policy • Donor eligibility

This article reconstructs governance practices related to blood policy that have developed within in the European Union (EU) over the last 15 years. It describes core aspects of the policy and argues that, despite an integrated cooperative approach between policy-makers and practitioners, this policy remains an open and evolving process. The European Blood Directive (2002/98/EC) and its subsequent directives managed, for the first time, to create an overarching framework for transfusion procedures. This framework consists of a number of standard definitions as well as detailed standard operating procedures (SOPs), yet leaves room for interpretation and different practices between EU member states. A recently published report on the progress of transposition of the Directives into national legislation reveals different standards, suggesting a lack of uniformity of safety and quality requirements. Further, gaps in the directives amount to practical medical problems, while increased mobility among EU citizens may add further problems to achieving the objective of a self-sufficient supply of blood and blood products. This might undermine public confidence in the quality of blood products and the health protection of donors, which, in turn, must be countered by a cooperative effort of policy-makers and blood establishments. Blood policies have been on the agenda of the European Community for more than 15 years. They pertain to both qualitative as well as quantitative issues; that is, assuring the quality and safety of blood and its derived products while simultaneously ensuring its availability in sufficient quantities. As early as 1994, the European Commission identified the need for a comprehensive strategy.[1,2] Voluntary, unpaid donations were meant to ensure self-sufficiency in blood and plasma, for which the

Faculty of Social Sciences and Economics, University of Hamburg, Allende Platz 1, Hamburg 20146, Germany
E-mail address: Hannes.Hansen-Magnusson@wiso.uni-hamburg.de

Clin Lab Med 30 (2010) 489–497
doi:10.1016/j.cll.2010.02.008
0272-2712/10/$ – see front matter © 2010 Elsevier Inc. All rights reserved.

Commission needed to learn about European citizens' perception and understanding of blood-related issues as well as citizens' attitude toward donating.

A survey among citizens of the EU revealed that "citizens are reasonably well-informed about general blood issues but several misconceptions do exist reflecting the need for further information and education programs about blood and plasma donation."[3] To this end, the report was meant to "be of value to national health authorities, blood collection and transfusion organizations, blood donor associations, and the plasma products industry in their efforts to contribute to achieving the goal of Community self-sufficiency in blood and plasma."[3]

The remainder of this article specifies how these objectives were meant to be achieved—yet how they remain an unfinished process. To this end, the article details the content of the European Blood Directive and some of its subsequent specifications that were meant to build an overarching framework across EU member states. It then sets out to analyze a recently published report on the transposition progress of the directives into national legislation. The report reveals that differences continue to exist between member states on a number of factors. Further problems on the road toward a safe and self-sufficient supply stem from gaps in the directives, causing medical problems, as well as from (potential) social and political developments. From these considerations, it can be concluded that despite the creation of blood directives at the EU level, the governance of blood remains an ongoing process and a site of construction.

BLOOD POLICY IN THE EU: DEVELOPING DIRECTIVE 2002/98/EC

In the aftermath of the 1995 survey, a concerted effort to ensure sufficient supplies was brought under way. It developed in cooperation between the European Commission as the authoritative norm-setter as well as the European Blood Alliance (EBA) that was founded in autumn 1998. The EBA consists of members "with a spectrum of organization arrangements ranging from the centrally managed national services (...) to local and regional services."[4] Their aim is to increase awareness in the public and among professionals as to the non-remunerated donation of blood and the preparation of its components for therapeutic purposes; to provide technical and professional support to members; and to develop facilities for and coordinate information-sharing on a national, European, and global level. In 2006, blood donations from EBA members' blood services amounted to around 15.5 million donations from a population of just over 300 million people.[4] For comparison, there were approximately 9.6 million allogeneic blood donors in the United States in the same year.[5] In the meantime, the EBA commented on and contributed expert advice to the European Blood Directive (EC/2002/98).

Directive 2002/98/EC and its Successors

The Blood Directive from 2002 was the first and groundbreaking attempt to devise uniform standards of quality and safety for human blood and its components. It did so by defining minimum safety criteria with a view to contributing to public confidence in terms of the quality of blood and blood products, as well as health protection of the donors. In line with the initial objectives of 1994, further intentions were to attain self-sufficiency and enhance confidence in the safety of the transfusion chain. The directive is binding for member states of the EU but it leaves open the choice of form and methods to comply, which includes the possibility of introducing more rigorous standards. Directive 2002/98/EC is termed the Mother Directive because it functions as a standard-setter while triggering further, more specific directives.

Following 2002/98/EC were three further directives that set out technical implementation measures for issues identified in the Mother Directive. Directive 2004/33/EC pertained to technical requirements for blood and blood components. Directive 2005/61/EC specified traceability requirements and requirements for the notification of serious adverse reactions and events. Finally, Directive 2005/62/EC provided standards and specifications relating to a quality system for blood establishments, similar to those established by the American Association of Blood Banks in the United States.[2] As Listl and Klouche[1] note, these directives were vital for the harmonization of European blood and blood-component comparability as well as transfer within Europe because they provided a catalog of definitions that did not exist previously. Either central terms were not clearly defined, or regulations did not exist in some member states.

An example of the specificity is provided by Seidl and colleagues[2] with regard to the quality system entailed in the Mother Directive and Directive 2005/62/EC. Regarding the former, they list the description of the quality system to include:

1. An organization chart, including responsibilities of responsible persons and reporting relationships
2. A site master file or quality manual describing the quality system in accordance with Article 11(1)
3. Number and qualifications of personnel
4. Hygienic provisions
5. Premises and equipment
6. List of SOPs for:
   Donor recruitment
   Retention and assessment of donors
   Processing and testing
   Distribution and recall of blood and blood components
   Reporting and recording of serious adverse reactions and events.

Specifications

On this basis, Directive 2005/62/EC sets out standards and specifications for blood establishments to ensure the safety of blood across Europe. Guidelines for a quality system were developed by a multinational project under the leadership of the German Red Cross Donor Service of Baden-Württemberg. The project entailed a consortium of sixteen members and established a project platform on the implementation of good practice. It developed a common format and regulations for SOPs to carry out an activity to demonstrate compliance with procedures,[2,6] supported by the EBA.

In the absence of absolute criteria, the quality management system developed is hierarchically structured in seven steps. They range from the framework of regulations via guidelines on document change control and personnel training to SOPs that are simple and user-friendly, listing precise quality requirements, requisites, and quality terms linked to the EU directives. At the same time, these standards cross-reference with or exist in addition to processes based on good manufacturing practice, good laboratory practice, and International Organization for Standardization (ISO) norms because blood establishments vary in size and often comprise several production sites. Such nexus of procedural regulations enables the compatibility of sites and eases exchange of supplies to external sites. The authors conclude that there is a list of benefits that includes:

- the definition of an overall quality policy
- improved personnel responsibility, qualification and training

- error and risk assessment system
- continuous improvement
- improved resource management
- performance improvement.[2]

Although the implementation process of quality control is complex, a positive cost effect is expected in the mid- to long-run, particularly if synergetic effects between the EU directives and good manufacturing practice and ISO standards can be exploited.[2,6]

THE IMPLEMENTATION PROCESS

In the run-up to a meeting of the competent blood authorities, attendees were asked to answer a "questionnaire on the transposition and implementation of the European regulatory framework of blood and blood components."[7] It was prepared before a meeting of competent blood authorities on January 29, 2009, comprising of EU member states, candidate countries (Croatia, Former Yugoslav Republic of Macedonia, and Turkey), and European Free Trade Association countries (Iceland, Liechtenstein, Norway, and Switzerland). The questionnaire was intended to determine whether countries had indeed transposed the four Directives into national law, reasons for a delay, and details regarding selected further issues. The report provides detailed information on:

- the national blood authority (name and address of national authority)
- transposition (has the transposition process been completed?)
- authorization (how many blood establishments are there in the country?)
- hospital blood banks (how many are there in the country?)
- inspections (is a system in place, how many inspections have been performed?)
- donor eligibility criteria (regarding exemption in accordance with Annex III.2.2.2 of Directive 2004/33/EC) (Annex III.2.2.2 of Directive 2004/33/EC: "Persons whose sexual behavior puts them at high risk of acquiring severe infectious diseases that can be transmitted by blood.")
- vigilance (serious adverse events and reactions)
- testing requirements
- imports and exports of blood and blood components
- sanctions (have authorizations been revoked or suspended, or have penalties been imposed?)
- others (eg, difficulties encountered in the transposition process).

The report may conclude the transposition process of the Directives but, based on the analysis of answers provided, it still leaves possibility for improving the safety of blood and blood derivates across Europe. On one hand, not all countries participating in the meeting in January 2009 provided full information on the sections above. At the time of publication on January 15, 2010 some empty spaces still had not been filled. This includes candidate and European Free Trade Association countries that are not obliged to comply with the Directives to an extent that member states must; but also some of the EU member states. On the other hand, the report also reveals that different criteria may exist across countries. This therefore leaves open the question whether blood is indeed of a uniform standard across the EU and its surrounding countries.

For instance, concerning donor eligibility criteria in EU member states for which a certain specification had to be provided, there are about four different answers.

Countries that provide a comprehensive account of exclusion criteria regarding risk-laden sexual behavior usually specify these as homosexual relations, heterosexual relations with changing partners, or unprotected intercourse, as well as intercourse for drugs or money, often in connection with prostitution. In addition, sometimes this risk group is expanded by excluding potential donors that have visited regions with a high rate of HIV or hepatitis. Countries that have expanded the sexual-practice deferral include Austria, Cyprus, Czech Republic, Denmark, France, Germany, Lithuania, the Netherlands, Slovenia, Sweden, and the United Kingdom. Romania forms a category by itself, listing the treatment for hemophilia before 1988 as the criterion for exclusion. A third group is formed by countries that answer affirmatively to whether exclusion criteria are in place (Finland, Greece, Hungary, Italy, Latvia, Luxembourg, Malta, Poland, and Portugal). Finally, Bulgaria, the Republic of Ireland, and Slovakia state that no national guidelines exist for the assessment of at risk sexual behaviors.

Table 1 provides a comprehensive overview of EU member states' testing requirements (excluding Estonia). The table reveals that there exists a consensual procedure for testing requirements for three infectious agents (hepatitis B surface antigen, anti-hepatitis C virus, and anti-HIV 1/2). However, apart from these three tests, member states proceed unilaterally. Some even demand further tests to be conducted, as specified in the table. Nonetheless, member states exchange blood if they have the necessary procedures in place, which usually refers to the existence of compatible safety standards in the country of origin, but may include regular on-site inspections such as Germany demands. The exception is the United Kingdom, which does not export blood or blood components because of variant Creutzfeldt-Jakob disease risks. The report does not specify whether the reason is that the United Kingdom refrains from exporting voluntarily or whether this is a consequence of EU member states refusing to import blood from the United Kingdom. The latter case might be the reason, judging from Germany's policy to deny donations from people who have spent more than 10 months in the United Kingdom between 1980 and 1996.

Apart from the special role of the United Kingdom, the EU forms a relatively closed market for blood and blood components. Trade of components within the EU takes place as long as bilateral agreements and comparable minimum standards exist. However, trade in blood and blood products is not necessarily well documented, meaning that there is usually a lack of data in terms of volumes exported (and, by implication, imported). Greece claims to have imported 26,000 units of blood cells from Switzerland, a non-EU member country, during 2008, while Sweden imports plasma used as a source material for medicinal products from the United States. On the other hand, Poland exported 107,032.5 L of plasma for fractionation to other EU countries while Germany exported 1,136,060 L of plasma for fractionation without specifying the destination. France exported 55 red blood cell concentrates and 6 fresh frozen plasmas to 13 countries (Algeria, Belgium, Canada, Congo, Egypt, Gabon, Germany, Hungary, Ireland, Mali, Nigeria, Senegal, and Switzerland).[7]

Possible Problems

The primary objective of the European Community was to establish a safe and reliable supply of blood and blood products to citizens across Europe. A European Blood Directive was developed and specified in cooperation with national and regional blood establishments in the subsequent years. This effort resulted in the Mother Directive of 2002 and three directives that specified its content. Again, in practice, the specific implementation arrangements were developed by practitioners, resulting inter alia in

Table 1
Testing requirements in EU member states

	Anti HBc	HBs ag	NAT HBV	Anti HCV	NAT HCV	Anti HIV-1/2	Ag HIV	NAT HIV 1	Treponema Pallidum	HTLV	Further Tests?
Austria	✓	✓	✓	✓	✓	✓		✓	✓		Nonspecific immunactivating marker (eg, neopterin)
Belgium		✓	✓	✓	✓	✓		✓	✓		Anti-HBc for new donors and on indication
Bulgaria		✓		✓		✓	✓		✓		
Cyprus	✓	✓	✓	✓	✓	✓	✓		✓		CMV for immunosuppressed patients
Czech Republic	✓	✓		✓		✓	✓		✓		
Denmark	✓	✓	✓	✓	✓	✓		✓		✓[a]	
Finland	✓	✓	✓	✓	✓	✓	✓	✓			According to the epidemiologic situation, extra testing may be required
France	✓	✓	✓	✓	✓	✓		✓	✓	✓	NAT HBV* In some French areas with particular epidemiologic situations (French overseas departments) Detection of malaria infectious markers. If necessary (individuals who have lived a malarial area or with history of undiagnosed febrile illness, visitors to endemic area)
Germany	✓	✓		✓	✓	✓	✓	✓	✓		
Greece	✓	✓	✓	✓	✓	✓	✓	✓	✓	✓	
Hungary	✓	✓		✓		✓			✓		
Rep. of Ireland	✓	✓		✓	✓	✓		✓			

Country									Additional tests / notes
Italy	✓	✓	✓	✓	✓	✓	✓	✓	
Latvia	✓	✓	✓	✓	✓	✓		✓	
Lithuania	✓	✓	✓	✓	✓	✓		✓	
Luxembourg	✓	✓	✓	✓	✓	✓		?	VDRL
Malta	✓	✓	✓	✓	✓	✓	✓	✓	Tests are required for: hemoglobin, liver function, anti-CMV/parvovirus (on request)
Netherlands	✓	✓	✓	✓	✓		✓	✓	Parvo B19 for selected donations and bacterial culture for all platelets
Poland	✓	✓	✓	✓	✓		✓	✓	ALT
Portugal	?	✓	✓	✓	✓	✓	✓	✓	
Romania	✓	✓	✓	✓	✓		✓	✓	HIV testing is performed using AG/antibody anti HIV combined kits
Slovakia	✓	✓	✓	✓	✓	✓	✓	✓	
Slovenia	?	✓	✓	✓	✓	✓	✓	?	NAT, anti HIV1/2/0 and p24Ag, HIV RNA, HCV RNA, HBV DNA are obligatory
Spain	✓	✓	✓	✓	✓		✓	✓	Trypanosoma cruzi
Sweden	✓	✓	✓	✓	✓		✓	✓	Hemoglobin
United Kingdom	✓	✓	✓	✓	✓		✓	✓	Not for mandatory donor screening. Certain additional tests may be performed, depending on need, eg, anti-CMV

Abbreviations: Ag, antigen; ALT, alanine aminotransferase; Anti, antibody; CMV, cytomegalovirus; HBc, hepatitis B core antigen; HBs, hepatitis B surface; HCV, hepatitis C virus; HTLV, human T-lymphotrophic virus; NAT, nucleic acid amplification technology.

^a Only first time donors.

From European Commission. Summary table of responses from competent authorities for blood and blood components. Questionnaire on the transposition and implementation of the European regulatory framework blood and blood components. Brussels, Health and Consumers Directorate-General; January 15, 2010.

SOP handbooks. Meanwhile, EU member states have gradually transposed the Directive into national legislation where it is now one of standards to ensure the quality of blood and its derivative products.

However, potential problems remain, pertaining to medical as well as political issues. On the medical side, an assessment of the implementation questionnaire reveals that different standards for testing requirements exist. Given that only three common transmissible disease-testing requirements can be found across member states, one wonders whether a uniform level of quality has been achieved. Another indicator toward this conclusion can be found in the very different amount of detail provided regarding data on import and export of blood and blood products between member states or across EU borders. In a similar vein, Listl and Klouche[1] state that Directive 2004/33/EC is not specific enough in terms of the required bacteriologic control, leaving the interpretation of the implication to member states.

The other, potentially more pressing, issue is political in nature. It concerns several points. First, there is the problem of growth. During the period of developing the different blood directives, the EU grew from 15 member states in 1995 to the current number of 27. During any growth process, accession candidates are required to accept the entire *acquis communautaire*, that is, the existing legal framework of the EU. This might be a source of concern as new members may not yet have transposed directives into national legislation and standards of safety might not be in operation. Consequently, the tradability and availability of blood and blood products might be hampered. Second, a concern arises from admission criteria that are closely linked to citizens' mobility throughout and out of the EU. As Listl and Klouche[1] write, criteria in Directive 2004/33/EC "lack explicit exclusion criteria for several relevant parasitic infectious diseases, eg, mucocutaneous leishmaniosis or trypanosomiasis, while other guidelines regarding for instance toxoplasmosis, do only apply to blood but not to plasma destined for fractionation. In view of the occurrence of some of these infectious diseases in certain European countries, the continuous presence of immigrants from endemic countries, and the extent of international travel, these risks may not have received sufficient attention."[8] Third, exclusion criteria might run counter to EU regulations that not only seek to promote mobility but also adhere to the principle of nondiscrimination. Although some countries have explicitly excluded certain risk groups from donation, as noted previously, a few member states have not. This might, one day, result in a ruling by the European Court of Justice. Fourth, related to the previous point, eventually certain criteria might reduce the pool of potential donors. Unforeseen risks may diminish the potential for interchangeability of blood and blood products, similar to the case of the United Kingdom that does not export because of the risk of variant Creutzfeldt-Jakob disease.

SUMMARY

These considerations amount to the insight that, despite the formulation of the European Blood Directive in 2002 and its subsequent implementation and specification, blood policies in the EU remain a work in progress. Social and political developments will require adjustments and specifications in the future. At the same time, policies need to be devised to maintain a pool of (reliable) donors. As much as barriers (read: exclusion criteria) might counteract this objective, a continuous effort into positively swinging public opinion toward donation seems needed. This is likely to involve both the European Commission and practitioner organizations such as the EBA in the near future.

ACKNOWLEDGMENTS

Research assistance from Torben Schenk and Ilyas Saliba is gratefully acknowledged.

REFERENCES

1. Listl S, Klouche M. The European Blood Directive (2002/98/EC) in the Context of the European Community Legislation. Transfus Med Hemother 2008;33:374–83.
2. Seidl C, O'Connell M, Delayney F, et al. European best practice in blood transfusion: improvement of quality-related processes in blood establishments. ISBT Science Series 2007;2(1):143–9.
3. European Commission. Europeans and Blood. Eurobarometer 41.0. Brussels: Directorate-General Employment Industrial Relations and General Affairs; 1995. p. 3.
4. Gorham M. Structure and governance of blood services: an European view. ISBT Science Series 2008;3(1):115–8.
5. U.S. Department of Health and Human Services. The 2007 National Blood Collection and Utilization Survey Report. Washington, DC: DHHS; 2007.
6. The project's website. Available at: http://www.eu-q-blood-sop.de. Accessed January 25, 2010.
7. European Commission. Summary table of responses from competent authorities for blood and blood components. Questionnaire on the transposition and implementation of the European regulatory framework blood and blood components [report]. Brussels: Health and Consumers Directorate-General; 2010.
8. Seidl C, Müller-Kuller T, Sireis W, et al. Levels of quality management of blood transfusion services in Europe. ISBT Science Series 2008;3(1):54–62.

Emerging Pathogens in Transfusion Medicine

Roger Y. Dodd, PhD

KEYWORDS

- Blood transfusion • Infectious disease
- Emerging infections • Blood safety

Transmission of infectious agents has long been recognized as an adverse outcome of transfusion, with the earliest concerns directed toward syphilis and viral hepatitis. Testing donors for evidence of syphilis infection was established in the 1940s, but in the absence of effective knowledge about viral hepatitis, the earliest measures relied on questioning of donors about a history of hepatitis: a precaution still in place, despite its currently demonstrable absence of value. The frequency of post-transfusion hepatitis prompted epidemiologic studies in the late 1950s, eventually leading to the elimination of blood collection from prison inmates and discouraging the use of paid donors. The essentially serendipitous discovery of HBsAg and of its relationship to hepatitis B opened up the use of donor testing but also revealed that another viral hepatitis (subsequently termed hepatitis C) was transmissible by transfusion. After a great deal of pioneering work, the causative agent (hepatitis C virus [HCV]) was identified by molecular techniques, antigens were expressed, and a test for antibodies to virus was developed and implemented for blood donors in 1990. Additionally, over the years, it became apparent that malaria could be transmitted by transfusion and deferral policies were established to prevent the collection of blood from individuals potentially exposed to malaria outside the United States. Taken together, these approaches, established for existing, chronic infections, defined the mechanisms for dealing with subsequent transfusion transmitted diseases.

EMERGING INFECTIONS

Before 1980, it was generally thought that the problem of infectious diseases had been solved, at least in the developed world. But the advent of AIDS, the appearance of other novel diseases in human populations, and the expansion of other known infections led to the now well-established concept of emerging infections. These have been defined as those infections whose incidence in humans has increased within the past

American Red Cross, Holland Laboratory, 15601, Crabbs Branch Way, Rockville, MD 20855, USA
E-mail address: dodd@usa.redcross.org

Clin Lab Med 30 (2010) 499–509
doi:10.1016/j.cll.2010.02.007
0272-2712/10/$ – see front matter © 2010 Elsevier Inc. All rights reserved.

labmed.theclinics.com

2 decades or threatens to increase in the near future. There are many reasons that infections emerge; these have been described elsewhere,[1] but some key factors include ecological disturbances (including climate change), changes in human behaviors, failure of disease and vector control, urbanization, population movement, and genetic change among disease agents. Often, these and other factors work in concert.

Many emerging infection are zoonoses and, although the transition from an animal to a human disease may involve many steps,[2] it may be rapid. Such a transition may be facilitated by genetic change, but this is not always the case. Once established in human populations, outbreaks may prove explosive and worldwide, as exemplified by SARS, which was caused by a previously unrecognized animal coronavirus that apparently first infected humans in Southern China.[3,4] Thereafter, it spread rapidly, apparently in part due to the rapid movement of infected individuals by jet aircraft.

It has become clear that some emerging infections may be transmitted by transfusion—this potential exists for any infectious agent that has an asymptomatic bloodborne phase. It has also become apparent that, although HIV, the first emerging infection to have a significant impact on blood safety, was chronic, parenterally and sexually transmissible, these characteristics did not all apply to subsequent transfusion transmissible emerging agents, such as variant Creutzfeldt-Jakob disease (vCJD), West Nile virus (WNV) and *Babesia*. Thus, although it is important to be prepared for emerging infections that threaten blood safety, it will never be possible to make an accurate determination of the next agent of concern. A framework can be built to establish readiness for such an event, however. One such attempt is a recent effort to catalog and prioritize agents of likely concern.[5]

HIV/AIDS

As discussed previously, HIV/AIDS was the first emerging infection to have a profound and unexpected effect on blood safety. It was first recognized as a syndrome of unusual opportunistic infections and a normally rare malignancy (Kaposi's sarcoma) among gay males, Haitian immigrants, drug abusers, and hemophiliacs. The etiology of the disease was unclear, although a leading hypothesis was that it was caused by an infectious agent. Eventually, a few cases were observed among individuals whose only potential risk factor was prior receipt of a blood transfusion.[6] Eventually, the etiologic agent was determined to be a retrovirus, now known as the human immunodeficiency virus (HIV), codiscovered by Montagnier and Gallo and their collaborators in 1983–1984.[7,8] By March of 1985, tests for antibodies to HIV had been developed and commercialized and their routine use for blood donations had been initiated.

It became apparent that the actual epidemic of HIV infection had started many years previously and that the disease itself had an extended incubation period, perhaps as long as 10 years. As a result, many individuals had unknowingly been infected and at least 12,000 transfusion transmissions had occurred in the United States alone.[9] This occurred in spite of measures that had been taken to defer donors with risk factors, in part because they had been implemented too late. Back-calculation showed that more than 1% of blood donations in San Francisco were probably infectious for AIDS at the beginning of the 1980s and that preventative measures resulted in a major decrease in that risk even before testing was put in place.[10] Because of the social sensitivity of the issues, early measures placed much reliance on education of donor populations and requests for self-deferral of those with risk factors, but within a few years, direct questioning of donors had been introduced. Even at the height of the epidemic, fewer that 2% of all AIDS cases in the United States were attributable to transfusion.

Shortly after the introduction of testing for HIV antibodies, it was found that nation-wide, approximately 0.038% of donors were seropositive; almost all of them would have been infectious. The majority of seropositive individuals were men with a history of having had sex with other men; this finding led to a tightening of donor questioning strategies.[11] Measures to reduce the risk of HIV transmission by transfusion have continued to be refined and tightened over the years, with increasing focus on: donor questioning; enhanced test sensitivity, including the addition of nucleic acid testing in 1999 (in the United States); and, now, interest in the implementation of pathogen reduction technology. The measures taken to date have proved efficacious: modeling studies suggest that the residual risk of transfusion transmission is on the order of 1 per 1.5 to 2 million component units in the United States, but the actual number of transmissions detected is much lower, with only 4 cases recognized in the United States between 1999 and 2009.

HIV/AIDS is widely recognized as an enormous human tragedy and it continues to be a devastating global epidemic. It undoubtedly had a profound impact on transfusion medicine, but it also materially affected and reoriented global attitudes toward blood safety. Before the advent of AIDS, there was a prevailing attitude that the development of some cases of post-transfusion infection was expected as an inevitable conse-quence of transfusion. This is not to say the issue was ignored, rather, that it was not an overriding priority. In several countries, those responsible for transfusion were subsequently held responsible for failing to prevent transmission of HIV/AIDS by trans-fusion and were actually prosecuted. In addition, many civil cases were brought against hospitals and blood centers on behalf of patients who had been infected. Whether or not these responses were appropriate will continue to be argued, but it is clear that there is now a low tolerance for failing to deal with any transfusion-transmitted infection. This may best be illustrated by the high cost-effectiveness ratio of many of the measures that have been routinely implemented in support of blood safety.

Although HIV/AIDS is now considered to be a globally endemic, rather than an emerging, infection, the virus itself is continuingly evolving. New clades and recombi-nant forms of the virus continue to appear, and there is justifiable concern that emer-gent subtypes may not be readily detectable by current test methods. This occurrence has already been observed, particularly with the type O clade, which emerged in some West African countries.[12,13] Continuing surveillance must be assured, along with monitoring of the capabilities of test kits to detect infection with new strains.

vCJD

Although there have been no cases of transmission of classical CJD by transfusion, the possibility has always been of concern, as exemplified by regulatory requirements around the disease. Also, transfusion transmission of animal-adapted strains has been shown in small animal models. When vCJD first appeared in humans (as a result of exposure to the BSE agent present in the food chain), there was concern that this new, emergent transmissible spongiform encephalopathy (TSE) might prove a risk to transfusion safety. This concern arose from the unknown nature of the infection and its unusual association with lymphoid cells and tissues. As a result, several preventative measures were put in place, well before there was any actual evidence of transfusion transmission. In the United States, the primary intervention was to defer as donors any individuals who had spent time in the United Kingdom at the peak of the BSE epidemic. The deferral was subsequently extended by including Western European countries (albeit with a different residence time) and eventually by deferring individuals receiving a blood transfusion in the United Kingdom. Several other criteria for deferral were also introduced; all are described on the Food and Drug Administraion Web site (http://www.fda.gov/BiologicsBloodVaccines/GuidanceComplianceRegulatoryInformation/Guidances/Blood/default.htm). In the United Kingdom, the deferral option was not available, but universal leukodepletion was introduced, locally derived plasma was no longer sent for fractionation, and plasma for transfusion was imported from countries at low risk of BSE.

As a result of careful surveillance, 4 cases of transmission of the vCJD agent by blood transfusion have been identified in England.[14,15] Three of the cases resulted in the development of fatal vCJD in recipients of blood that was collected from donors who subsequently developed vCJD. In a fourth instance, the agent was found in the spleen and 1 lymph node of a similarly exposed but asymptomatic individual who died of unconnected causes. The source of the infection was a donor who had transmitted the disease to 1 of the other 3 cases. All of these cases were attributable to blood components that had not been leukoreduced. More recently, the agent was also identified at autopsy in a hemophilia patient who had received products from plasma pools that included units thought to be at risk of containing the agent (http://www.hpa.org.uk/webw/HPAweb&HPAwebStandard/HPAweb_C/1234859690542?p=1231252394302). The agent has also been shown to be transmissible in a sheep model.[16]

At the time of this writing, the small epidemic of vCJD seems to be declining, although there is some concern that there may be future waves of disease among individuals with a genotype that differs from the one seen in almost all clinical cases of vCJD to date. Further, management of the food chain has reduced or eliminated the risk of food-borne exposure to BSE. In these circumstances, the need for further interventions may be arguable. This would be the case in the United States, where there do not yet seem to be any cases of locally acquired vCJD. Nevertheless, 2 companies have developed and CE-marked affinity based systems for removal of TSE prions from red cell concentrates.[17,18] One of them has been evaluated in the United Kingdom and Ireland.

WNV

In 1999, a small outbreak of West Nile virus infection occurred in Queens, New York. This was the first reported occurrence of this flavivirus in the Western Hemisphere. It is not known how the virus was introduced into the United States, although it undoubtedly involved rapid intercontinental transportation. Perhaps unexpectedly, the virus rapidly spread across the continent, infecting hundreds of thousands of individuals.[19] Although the resulting infections were acute, modeling studies suggested that transfusion transmission of WNV was possible and shortly after the first such study was published in 2002,[20] 23 transfusion transmissions were reported.[21] As a result of an exemplary cooperation between manufacturers, transfusion medicine specialists, public health authorities, and regulators, tests for WNV RNA were developed, commercialized and implemented within less than 1 year. The strategy has been successful, although it is not possible to prevent all infections solely by the use of pooled testing: conversion to single donation testing is necessary in times and places with high incidence rates for infection. Careful implementation of this strategy has been shown to eliminate residual infections, at least in 1 large blood system.

The emergence of WNV in the United States and the finding that it was transmissible by transfusion did challenge preconceived notions. First, that the most likely new concern to blood safety would come from an agent with epidemiologic characteristics similar to those of HBV and HIV, and second, that acute infections would offer only minimal risk of transfusion transmission. It also illustrated the fact that a test for nucleic acids is relatively easy to develop and implement in a short time -frame.[22] It also led to the recognition that other arboviruses might behave in the same way as WNV, by causing unexpected large outbreaks, consequently compromising blood safety. As discussed later, there have been recent examples illustrating this concern, involving dengue and chikunguya viruses.

Chagas Disease

In contrast to WNV, *T cruzi*, the parasitic agent of Chagas disease, entered the US population as a result of gradual immigration. The majority of infected individuals identified in the United States were born in Latin American countries in which the parasite is endemic. Infection usually occurs early in life and is essentially lifelong, with the potential for late clinical outcomes, cardiac or digestive.Parasite and competent insect vectors, however, do exist naturally in most of the southern US states, even though transmission to humans is uncommon in the United States.

T cruzi has long been recognized as transmissible by transfusion, and in most Latin American countries, donor testing for antibodies to the parasite is routine.[23,24] There have been 7 documented cases of transmission in the United States and Canada, and in all cases where the origins of the infection could be determined, it derived from platelets donated by an individual who had been born, or was a resident in, South America. Extended research studies showed that a significant proportion of blood donors, particularly in California and Florida, were infected with *T cruzi*.[25] A test for antibodies to *T cruzi* was licensed in the United States in late 2006 and was implemented at the beginning of 2007. Nationwide, the donor prevalence rate was found to be approximately 1:30,000.[26] Some of the seropositive donors did not have geographic risk factors and seemed to have been infected in the United States. Lookback studies on prior recipients of blood from seropositive donors, however, revealed only 2 infections from a total of 241 recipients examined (http://www.fda.gov/AdvisoryCommittees/CommitteesMeetingMaterials/ BloodVaccinesandOtherBiologics/BloodProductsAdvisoryCommittee/ucm155529. htm). This was 1 of the factors that led to a reevaluation of the value of testing and consideration of selective testing strategies. Such strategies were discussed at a meeting of the FDA's Blood Products Advisory Committee. The Committee endorsed the concept of selective testing, specifically on the basis of testing each donor once and accepting seronegative donors without need for any futher testing. The Committtee did, however, express concern abut the possibility of incident (new) infections among donors and recommended that selective testing be considered only if a continuing study of incidence of *T cruzi* infection among donors was to be conducted. One major blood supplier in the United States implemented selective (1-time) testing in August 2009 and several other smaller establishments used a variety of alternate approaches to selective testing.

Babesia

Babesia is a malaria-like, intraerythrocytic protozoan parasite that is transmitted by ticks. In the United States, the predominant species is *B microti*, which is transmitted by Ixodid ticks, particularly *I scapularis*. There are particular foci of infection in the coastal areas of New England and in the upper Midwest. The parasite may be regarded as emerging, as it seems that its range is expanding and that opportunities for human infection are also increasing.[27] Other species of *Babesia* have been identified in Missouri, California, and Washington. The parasite is readily transmitted from infected donors by transfusion and more than 70 such cases have been documented in the United States: some have been fatal.[28,29] The risk of infection is high in areas of greatest endemicity, perhaps exceeding 1:1000 in parts of Connecticut. Some donors may be infected and infectious for periods of 6 months or more.

Effective interventions against transfusion transmitted babesiosis do not currently exist. A licensed test is not available nor is an appropriate donor questioning strategy. Some blood establishments avoid collections from areas of high endemicity during the tick season, but given the potentially prolonged period of infectivity, such a strategy is not fully effective. Furthermore, donors and their blood may travel and several transfusion transmissions have occurred in areas that are not endemic for Babesia. There is increasing concern about Babesia and blood transfusion in the United States, as illustrated by an FDA-sponsored workshop held September 12, 2008 (http://www.fda.gov/BiologicsBloodVaccines/NewsEvents/WorkshopsMeetingsConferences/TranscriptsMinutes/default.htm), but the future path is currently unclear. It seems most likely that some geographically limited testing will eventually be implemented for blood donations.

EMERGING INFECTIONS OF POTENTIAL CONCERN FOR THE FUTURE

As discussed previously, it is not possible to predict which infections will emerge, or, once emerged, the extent to which they will compromise blood safety. Consequently, any discussion of specific agents must be regarded as speculative. Furthermore, outcomes may be geographically variable. For example, the pattern of emergence and human disease seen in the WNV outbreak is different from that seen in southern Europe. Further, although the virus is now present in the Caribbean and Central and South America, it does not seem to have the same impact on human health in those parts of the world as it has in North America.

Arboviruses

Until WNV emerged in the United States, arboviruses had not been seriously considered in the context of blood safety. Two of them, dengue (DENV) and chikungunya virus (CHIKV), have now attracted considerable attention, however. Although one is flavivirus and the other an alphavirus, they share common transmission patterns (human-mosquito-human) and vectors (Aedes aegypti and A albopictus). Both viruses cause large outbreaks of infection and disease and one of them has been shown to be transmissible by transfusion. It should also be noted that another flavivirus , St Louis encephalitis virus is endemic to the United States and has, in the past, been responsible for sporadic, but large outbreaks. Thus, it is reasonable to consider this agent to be a potential future threat: continuing surveillance is appropriate.

More specifically, 2 clusters of transfusion transmitted DENV have been reported, 1 from Hong Kong and 1 from Singapore.[30,31] A third transmission has been discussed but not yet published. Investigation of blood donor samples from Honduras, Brazil, and Puerto Rico has revealed significant frequencies of viremia during DENV outbreaks[32,33]; in 1 of these studies, not only have high titers of virus been demonstrated but also the viruses have been shown to be infectious in laboratory systems.[33] To date, there has been no standardized response by blood organizations to the issue of transfusion-transmissible DENV. Perhaps the most comprehensive reaction has been that of the Australian Red Cross Blood Services, which has routinely stopped collection of blood components for transfusion in parts of Northern Queensland during dengue outbreaks. If an intervention is judged necessary, it would be appropriate to consider the use of a test for DENV RNA: a measure comparable to that used for WNV. Such a test is not commercially available (at least as of early 2010), but a test for a viral NS1 antigen is available[34]; it would be expected to identify high-titer viremic donations.

CHIKV is normally endemic in East Africa, but over the past few years, has been responsible for several explosive epidemics, most notably (but not exclusively) in the Indian Ocean islands.[35] A factor that seemed to contribute was a viral mutation resulting in preferential transmission of the virus by the widely distributed *A albopictus* mosquito.[36] The outbreak in la Réunion has been particularly well described. Hundreds of thousands of residents, representing more than 40% of the population were infected. The island is an overseas department of France, and authorities took extensive steps to protect the safety of the blood supply. Tests for CHIKV nucleic acids were implemented (finding 2 in 500 donations to be viremic); red cell collections were discontinued on the island (needed red cells were provided directly from France); and pathogen reduction technology was implemented for platelet concentrates, which were collected locally.[37] Another small but unexpected outbreak occurred in Italy, as a result of an infected traveler.[38] This event also led to regional prohibition of blood collection for the duration of the outbreak.

Given this background, it is reasonable to speculate on the possible implications to other parts of the world, such as North America. As discussed previously, dengue is already endemic in Puerto Rico and is subject to annual outbreaks. There have also been outbreaks in Hawaii and a high seroprevalence rate has been found in residents of Brownsville, Texas, with much higher rates across the Mexican border. In late 2009, there was an outbreak of locally transmitted dengue in Key West (http://www.doh. state.fl.us/Environment/medicine/arboviral/Dengue_FloridaKeys.html). Certainly, *A aegypti* (the preferred vector for DENV) is present in parts of the Southern United States; thus, conditions exist for some spread of the virus on the mainland. It is not, however, clear that sustained transmission could occur. The issue for chikungunya may be a little more complex, as *A albopictus* is much more widespread and chikungunya cases among travelers returning to the United States are not uncommon.[39] There are many other arboviruses, but there is really no clear basis for making any predictions about their future spread.

TSEs

Experience with vCJD has been salutary. To date, there is no evidence that (despite animal model studies) classic CJD has been transmitted by transfusion. Lookback studies on recipients of blood from donors who subsequently developed CJD have been uniformly negative and show that, if such transmission is possible, it would be much less frequent than for vCJD.[40] Chronic wasting disease (CWD), an affliction of cervids in the United States, seems to be emerging. Given that it sems transmissible between animals by the oral route, it is reasonable to question whether or not it could become a human pathogen in a fashion analogous to BSE.[41] Despite some apparent clusters of CJD in younger individuals with a history of hunting,[42] there has been no evidence to date to support such a species jump for the CWD agent.

Retroviruses

As discussed previously, there is little doubt that the emergence of HIV/AIDS as a transfusion transmissible disease has materially altered perceptions about blood safety. In a more particular sense, it has also focused concern on retroviruses themselves. Two examples are relevant. The first is simian foamy virus, which has been shown to be transmissible to humans, generally as a result of close contact with monkeys in a professional or recreational (travel) setting.[43,44] To date, there has been no evidence whatever that such human infection has any clinical outcomes. Regulatory agencies, however, have questioned whether or not there might be risk of emergence of a pathogenic mutant of SFV in association with species jump.

When linked with concern about the potential for transfusion transmission of the virus (which has been demonstrated in macaques but not in humans),[45–48] this has led regulators to ask whether or not some intervention is warranted. Although such a proposal was not supported by the BPAC in the United States, Canadian regulators have imposed deferral from blood donation on individuals employed as monkey handlers.[49]

There has been renewed interest in the xenotropic murine leukemia-like retrovirus (XMRV) as a result of a high-profile article describing a potential association of this virus with chronic fatigue syndrome.[50] The article also suggested that evidence of XMRV infection could be found in 3.7% of normal controls and that the virus from the clinical cases was infectious in vitro. The authors of the publication expressed concern that the virus might be transmissible by transfusion[50]; a point also raised in an accompanying editorial. To date, however, there are no specific data to support this contention nor is there any current evidence that XMRV is the causative agent of any disease although it had previously been found in association with selected cases of prostate cancer. Studies will be planned to determine whether or not the virus is transmitted by transfusion.

PATHOGEN REDUCTION

Several interventions might be used to eliminate or reduce the risk of transfusion transmission of an emerging infection. They include measures based on management of donations in affected areas, donor medical, travel or risk history, implementation of tests, or product manipulation. None of these approaches is 100% effective, and all suffer from some disadvantages, such as poor sensitivity or specificity, lengthy development process, high direct or indirect costs, and so forth. Conceptually, it would be desirable to have a generic method that would be proactive instead of reactive. Many believe that pathogen inactivation represents such a solution. Several treatment methods are available for plasma for transfusion and for platelet concentrates but no method for red cell concentrates has yet been brought to market.[5] The approaches have been put into practice at least in part, in several European countries. Although the methods have been shown to effectively inactivate significant titers of a variety of pathogens and model organisms in laboratory studies, their potential for elimination of as yet unknown emerging infections is necessarily unknown. Also, the absence of methods that can inactivate all blood components is a disadvantage. It is also apparent that currently available methods do have some negative impact upon treated products. No method is currently available for use in the United States and the regulatory barrier appears to be high. Available methods, their properties and advantages and disadvantages are described in several reviews and other publications.[5,51,52]

REFERENCES

1. Weiss RA, McMichael AJ. Social and environmental risk factors in the emergence of infectious diseases. Nat Med 2004;10:S70–6.
2. Wolfe ND, Dunavan CP, Diamond J. Origins of major human infectious diseases. Nature 2007;447:279–83.
3. Guan Y, Zheng BJ, He YQ, et al. Isolation and characterization of viruses related to the SARS coronavirus from animals in southern China. Science 2003;302:276–8.
4. Vijayanand P, Wilkins E, Woodhead M. Severe acute respiratory syndrome (SARS): a review. Clin Med 2004;4:152–60.
5. Stramer SL, Hollinger FB, Katz LM, et al. Emerging infectious disease agents and their potential threat to transfusion safety. Transfusion. 2009;49(Suppl 2):1S–29S.

6. Peterman TA, Jaffe HW, Feorino PM, et al. Transfusion-associated acquired immunodeficiency syndrome in the United States. JAMA 1985;254:2913–7.

7. Barre-Sinoussi F, Chermann J-C, Rey F, et al. Isolation of a T-lymphotropic retrovirus from a patient at risk for acquired immune deficiency syndrome (AIDS). Science 1983;220:868–71.

8. Gallo RC, Salahuddin SZ, Popovic M, et al. Frequent detection and isolation of cytopathic retroviruses (HTLV-III) from patients with AIDS and at risk for AIDS. Science 1984;224:500–3.

9. Peterman TA, Lui K-J, Lawrence DN, et al. Estimating the risks of transfusion-associated acquired immune deficiency syndrome and human immunodeficiency virus infection. Transfusion 1987;27:371–4.

10. Busch MP, Young MJ, Samson SM, et al. Risk of human immunodeficiency virus (HIV) transmission by blood transfusions before the implementation of HIV-1 antibody screening. Transfusion 1991;31:4–11.

11. Schorr JB, Berkowitz A, Cumming PD, et al. Prevalence of HTLV-III antibodies in American blood donors. N Engl J Med 1985;313:384–5.

12. Apetrei C, Loussert-Ajaka I, Descamps D, et al. Lack of screening test sensitivity during HIV-1 non-subtype B seroconversions. AIDS 1996;10:F57–60.

13. Schable C, Zekeng L, Pau C-P, et al. Sensitivity of United States HIV antibody tests for detection of HIV-1 group O infections. Lancet 1994;344:1333–4.

14. Hewitt PE, Llewelyn CA, Mackenzie J, et al. Creutzfeldt-Jakob disease and blood transfusion: results of the UK Transfusion Medicine Epidemiological Review study. Vox Sang 2006;91:221–30.

15. Zou S, Fang CT, Schonberger LB. Transfusion transmission of human prion diseases. Transfus Med Rev 2008;22:58–69.

16. Houston F, McCutcheon S, Goldmann W, et al. Prion diseases are efficiently transmitted by blood transfusion in sheep. Blood 2008;112:4739–45.

17. Sowemimo-Coker SO, Pesci S, Andrade F, et al. Pall leukotrap affinity prion-reduction filter removes exogenous infectious prions and endogenous infectivity from red cell concentrates. Vox Sang 2006;90:265–75.

18. Gregori L, Gurgel PV, Lathrop JT, et al. Reduction in infectivity of endogenous transmissible spongiform encephalopathies present in blood by adsorption to selective affinity resins. Lancet 2006;368:2226–30.

19. Petersen LR, Hayes EB. Westward ho?—The spread of West Nile virus. N Engl J Med 2004;351:2257–9.

20. Biggerstaff BJ, Petersen LR. Estimated risk of West Nile virus transmission through blood transfusion during an epidemic in Queens, New York City. Transfusion 2002;42:1019–26.

21. Pealer LN, Marfin AA, Petersen LR, et al. Transmission of West Nile virus through blood transfusion in the United States in 2002. N Engl J Med 2003;349:1236–45.

22. Dodd RY. Emerging infections, transfusion safety, and epidemiology. N Engl J Med 2003;349:1205–6.

23. Schmuñis GA. Trypanosoma cruzi, the etiologic agent of Chagas' disease: status in the blood supply in endemic and nonendemic countries. Transfusion 1991;31:547–57.

24. Schmunis GA, Cruz JR. Safety of the blood supply in Latin America. Clin Microbiol Rev 2005;18:12–29.

25. Leiby DA, Read EJ, Lenes BA, et al. Seroepidemiology of Trypanosoma cruzi, etiologic agent of Chagas' disease, in US blood donors. J Infect Dis 1997;176:1047–52.

26. Bern C, Montgomery SP, Katz L, et al. Chagas disease and the US blood supply. Curr Opin Infect Dis 2008;21:476–82.
27. Leiby DA. Babesiosis and blood transfusion: flying under the radar. Vox Sang 2006;90:157–65.
28. Gubernot DM, Lucey CT, Lee KC, et al. Babesia infection through blood transfusions: reports received by the US Food and Drug Administration, 1997–2007. Clin Infect Dis 2009;48:25–30.
29. Tonnetti L, Eder AF, Dy B, et al. Transfusion-transmitted Babesia microti identified through hemovigilance. Transfusion 2009;49:2557–63.
30. Chuang VW, Wong TY, Leung YH, et al. Review of dengue fever cases in Hong Kong during 1998 to 2005. Hong Kong Med J 2008;14:170–7.
31. Tambyah PA, Koay ES, Poon ML, et al. Dengue hemorrhagic fever transmitted by blood transfusion. N Engl J Med 2008;359:1526–7.
32. Linnen JM, Vinelli E, Sabino EC, et al. Dengue viremia in blood donors from Honduras, Brazil, and Australia. Transfusion 2008;48:1355–62.
33. Mohammed H, Linnen JM, Munoz-Jordan JL, et al. Dengue virus in blood donations, Puerto Rico, 2005. Transfusion 2008;48:1348–54.
34. Kumarasamy V, Wahab AH, Chua SK, et al. Evaluation of a commercial dengue NS1 antigen-capture ELISA for laboratory diagnosis of acute dengue virus infection. J Virol Methods 2007;140:75–9.
35. Charrel RN, de L X, Raoult D. Chikungunya outbreaks—the globalization of vectorborne diseases. N Engl J Med 2007;356:769–71.
36. Tsetsarkin KA, Vanlandingham DL, McGee CE, et al. A single mutation in chikungunya virus affects vector specificity and epidemic potential. PLoS Pathog 2007; 3:e201.
37. Brouard C, Bernillon P, Quatresous I, et al. Estimated risk of Chikungunya viremic blood donation during an epidemic on Reunion Island in the Indian Ocean, 2005 to 2007. Transfusion 2008;48:1333–41.
38. Rezza G, Nicoletti L, Angelini R, et al. Infection with chikungunya virus in Italy: an outbreak in a temperate region. Lancet 2007;370:1840–6.
39. Lanciotti RS, Kosoy OL, Laven JJ, et al. Chikungunya virus in US travelers returning from India, 2006. Emerg Infect Dis 2007;13:764–7.
40. Dorsey K, Zou S, Schonberger LB, et al. Lack of evidence of transfusion transmission of Creutzfeldt-Jakob disease in a US surveillance study. Transfusion 2009; 49:977–84.
41. Belay ED, Maddox RA, Williams ES, et al. Chronic wasting disease and potential transmission to humans. Emerg Infect Dis 2004;10:977–84.
42. Belay ED, Gambetti P, Schonberger LB, et al. Creutzfeldt-Jakob disease in unusually young patients who consumed venison. Arch Neurol 2001;58:1673–8.
43. Jones-Engel L, Engel GA, Schillaci MA, et al. Primate-to-human retroviral transmission in Asia. Emerg Infect Dis 2005;11:1028–35.
44. Switzer WM, Bhullar V, Shanmugam V, et al. Frequent simian foamy virus infection in persons occupationally exposed to nonhuman primates. J Virol 2004;78: 2780–9.
45. Brooks JI, Merks HW, Fournier J, et al. Characterization of blood-borne transmission of simian foamy virus. Transfusion 2007;47:162–70.
46. Khan AS, Kumar D. Simian foamy virus infection by whole-blood transfer in rhesus macaques: potential for transfusion transmission in humans. Transfusion 2006;46:1352–9.
47. Boneva RS, Grindon AJ, Orton SL, et al. Simian foamy virus infection in a blood donor. Transfusion 2002;42:886–91.

48. Winkler IG, Flügel RM, Asikainen K, et al. Antibody to human foamy virus not detected in individuals treated with blood products or in blood donors. Vox Sang 2000;79:118–9.

49. O'Brien SF, Yi QL, Fearon MA, et al. A predonation screening question for occupational exposure to simian foamy virus: a preliminary donor survey in Canada. Transfusion 2007;47:949–50.

50. Lombardi VC, Ruscetti FW, Das GJ, et al. Detection of an infectious retrovirus, XMRV, in blood cells of patients with chronic fatigue syndrome. Science 2009; 326:585–9.

51. Prowse C, Robinson AE. Pathogen inactivation of labile blood components. Transfus Med 2001;11:147.

52. Webert KE, Cserti CM, Hannon J, et al. Proceedings of a Consensus Conference: pathogen inactivation-making decisions about new technologies. Transfus Med Rev 2008;22:1–34.

Index

Note: Page numbers of article titles are in **boldface** type.

A

Alloimmunization, to transfused blood products, **467–473**
    nonantibody-based immune responses, 469–471
    risk factors for, 468–469
American Rare Donor Program, 427
American trypanosomiasis, 503
Anemia
    hemolytic
        fetal blood group testing for, **431–442**
        warm autoimmune, 424–425
    preoperative correction of, 455, 457
Anticoagulants, for blood salvage, 459
Antigens
    absence of, in universal donor cells, 398–399, 445
    alloimmunization and, **467–473**
    alteration of, for universal donor red blood cell products, 445
    fetal, blood group testing for, **431–442**
    molecular testing for, **419–429**
        application of, 424–426
        automation of, 426
        costs of, 423–424
        data management for, 426–427
        polymorphism detection, 419–423
    pig blood, 367–369
Arboviruses, 504–505
Automation, of red blood cell genotyping, 426

B

Babesia, 503–504
Bead chip microarray analysis, for red blood cell genotyping, 422
Bioreactors, for stem cell processes, 409–413
Blood management, **453–465**
    conservation strategies for
        blood salvage in, 458–460
        normovolemic hemodilution in, 457–458
        point of care testing in, 460–462
        preoperative anemia prevention in, 455, 457
        program components in, 455–456
    definition of, 454–455
    impetus for, 453–454

Blood Products Advisory Committee, red blood cell recovery methods of, 444
Blood salvage, 458–460
Blood substitutes, **381–389**
   biochemical engineering of, 382–384
   biologic activity of, 384–386
   potency of, 384–386
   toxicity of, 386–387
   versus cells derived from stem cells, 392
Blood transfusion
   alloimmunization to, **467–473**
   antigen testing for, **419–429**
   avoidance or reduction of, **381–389, 453–465**
   blood management and, **453–465**
   blood supply for, 453–454
   costs of, 453
   European Blood Directive for, **489–497**
   fetal blood grouping for, **431–442**
   future status of, **405–417**
      drivers of change for, 406–408
      genetically engineered pigs and, 372–375
      red blood cell enrichment for, 413–414
      regulatory considerations in, 414–415
      stem cells in. *See* Stem cell(s).
   genetically engineered pigs for, **365–380**
   history of, 405–406
   need for, 406–407
   pathogens in, 407, **499–509**
   platelet storage lesion due to, **475–487**
   products for, **443–452**
   stem cell transformation for. *See* Stem cell(s).
   substitutes for, **381–389**
BLOODchip, for red blood cell genotyping, 421–422
"Bloodless Center," 454
Bone marrow transplantation, after alloimmunization to blood products, 470
Bovine spongiform encephalopathy, 501–502

C

C antigens, fetal testing for, 437
CD34 stem cells, red blood cells derived from, 408–411
Cellular transfusion products, **443–452**
   platelets, 446–449
   red blood cells, 444–446
Chagas disease, 503
Chikungunya virus, 504–505
Chronic wasting disease, 505
Contamination
   of blood products
      alloimmunization and, 468–469
      reduction of, 446–447
   of salvaged blood, 460

Creutzfeldt-Jakob disease, variant, 501–502
Critical Path Initiative, 449
Culture, of stem cells, for red blood cell production, 391–403, 408–415

D

D antigen, fetal testing for, 431–437
Data management, for red blood cell genotyping, 425–426
DCLHb blood substitute, 383
Dengue virus, 504–505
Donors
    European Blood Directive policy for, 489–497
    screening of, for rare phenotypes, 425

E

E antigens, fetal testing for, 437
Erythrocytes. *See* Red blood cells.
Erythropoiesis-stimulating agents, for preoperative anemia, 455, 457
European Blood Directive, **489–497**
    development of, 490–492
    implementation of, 492–496
    testing requirements of, 493–495

F

Fetal blood group testing, **431–442**
    D phenotype, 432–437
    maternal plasma for, 431–432
    non-D groups, 437–438
    quality assurance for, 438
FiberCell Systems, bioreactors of, 411–412
Food and Drug Administration, blood product standards of, 443–449
Free radical formation, in blood substitutes, 386–387

G

Gal epitope, in pig blood, 367–368
Genotyping, of red blood cells, **419–429**
Geron Corp., stem cell studies of, 409

H

HbDex blood substitute, 383
HEA microarray analysis, for red blood cell genotyping, 422
HemoCue hemoglobin analyzer, 461–462
Hemodilution, acute normovolemic, 457–458
Hemoglobin, generation of, in red blood cells derived from stem cells, 396
Hemoglobin-based oxygen carriers
    biochemical engineering of, 382–384
    biologic activity of, 384–386

Hemoglobin-based (*continued*)
    potency of, 384–386
    toxicity of, 386–387
    versus cells derived from stem cells, 392
Hemolink, 383–384
Hemolytic anemia
    fetal blood group testing for, **431–442**
    warm autoimmune, 424–425
Hemopure, 383
HIV/AIDS, 500–501
Human immunodeficiency virus, 500–501
Human leukocyte antigens, alloimmunization and, 469–470
Humoral immunization, to transfused blood products, 468–469
Hypoxia-inducible factor, 385

I

Iron-deficiency anemia, preoperative correction of, 455, 457

K

Kell antigens, fetal testing for, 437

L

LifeBank USA, stem cell studies of, 409
Luminex system, for red blood cell genotyping, 422–423

M

Mad cow disease, 501–502
Major histocompatibility complex, alloimmunization and, 469–470
Mass spectrometry
    for fetal blood group testing, 434, 438
    for red blood cell genotyping, 422–423
Matrix-assisted laser desorption ionization time of flight, for D antigen, 434, 438
Melting-curve analysis, for red blood cell genotyping, 421
Methoxy-polyethylene glycol, for red cell camouflage, 375
Microarray analysis, for red blood cell genotyping, 421–422
Myelodysplastic syndrome, 398

N

NeuGc epitope, in pig blood, 367–368
Nitric oxide, blood substitute interactions with, 386–387

O

OpenArray, for red blood cell genotyping, 422–423
Oxidants, in blood substitutes, 386–387
Oxygen carriers, hemoglobin-based, **381–389**

Oxygen equilibrium curves, of blood substitutes, 384–386
Oxyhemoglobin, 383

P

Pathogens, **499–509**
    arboviruses, 504–505
    Babesia, 503–504
    Chagas disease, 503
    HIV/AIDS, 500–501
    in platelet products, 447, 483
    in red blood cell products, 445–446
    problems with, 407
    retroviruses, 505–506
    transmissible spongiform encephalopathy, 501–502, 505
    variant Creutzfeldt-Jakob disease, 501–502
    West Nile virus, 502–503
Peroxidation, in blood substitutes, 387
Phenotype matching, 424–425
Pigs, genetically engineered, red blood cells from, **365–380**
    future of, 372–375
    history of, 366
    immunologic barriers and, 367–369
    polyethylene glycol-coated, 375
    primate studies of, 369–372
    similarity to human cells, 366–367
Platelet(s)
    degranulation of, tests for, 477
    morphology of, tests for, 477
    products containing
        characterization of, 476–478
        cold storage of, 446–447
        evaluation of, 448–449
        in vitro versus in vivo studies of, 478–481
        novel technologies for, 483–484
        pathogen reduction in, 447
        production of, 476
        shelf-life problems with, 475–476
        stem cell-derived, 448
        substitutes for, 447–448
        transfusion outcome and, 482–482
        viability tests for, 479–480
Platelet additive solutions, 483
Platelet storage lesion, **475–487**
Pluripotent stem cells, red blood cells derived from, 399
Point of care testing, in blood management, 460–462
Polymerase chain reaction
    for D antigen, 434
    for red blood cell genotyping, 420–422
Polymorphisms, of red blood cells, detection of, 419–423
Prions, 501–502
Pyrosequencing, for red blood cell genotyping, 421

Q

Quality assurance, for fetal blood group testing, 438

R

Red blood cells
   antigens of. *See* Antigens.
   from genetically engineered pigs, **365–380**
   from stem cell transformation. *See* Stem cell(s).
   genotyping of, **419–429**
      application of, 424–426
      automation of, 426
      costs of, 423–424
      data management for, 426–427
   hemoglobin-based oxygen carriers prepared from, 382–384
   products containing, 444–446
      evaluation of, 444, 448–449
      pathogen reduction in, 445–446
      shelf life extension for, 445
      storage of, 444–445
      universal donor, 445
Regulations
   for red blood cell transformation, 414–415
   in European Blood Directive, **489–497**
Rejection, of products, 470
Reticulocytes, maturation and conservation of, 394, 396
Retroviruses, 505–506
RhD blood group, fetal testing for, 431–437

S

Salvage, of blood, 458–460
Sickle cell disease, 398
Simian foamy virus, 505–506
SNaPshot system, for red blood cell genotyping, 422
SNPstream system, for red blood cell genotyping, 422
Stem cell(s)
   platelets derived from, 448
   red blood cells derived from, **391–403**
      candidates for, 398
      differentiation of, 396, 413–414
      enrichment strategies for, 413–414
      for universal red blood cells, 398–399
      future of, 400–402
      industrial scale process for, 399–400
      large-scale processes for, 409–413
      lifespan study for, 397
      marketing of, 400
      maturation of, 394–396
      need for, 391–393

novel bioreactors for, 409–413
pluripotent, 399
potential of, 408–409
proliferation in, 393–394
quantitative aspect of, 397
regulatory considerations in, 414–415
simplification of procedure for, 396–397
Stem Cell Systems, bioreactors of, 412–413
Storage
    of platelet products, 446–447, **475–487**
    of red blood cell products, 444–445
Substitutes, for blood, **381–389**
Swirl test, for platelet products, 478

T

Transfusion, blood. *See* Blood transfusion.
Transmissible spongiform encephalopathy, 501–502, 505
Transplantation, after alloimmunization to blood products, 469–471
Trypanosoma cruzi, 503

U

Universal donor red blood cells, 398–399, 445

W

West Nile virus, 502–503

X

Xenotransfusions, from genetically engineered pigs, **365–380**
Xenotropic murine leukemia-like retrovirus, 506

Moving?

Make sure your subscription moves with you!

To notify us of your new address, find your **Clinics Account Number** (located on your mailing label above your name), and contact customer service at:

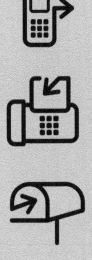

Email: journalscustomerservice-usa@elsevier.com

800-654-2452 (subscribers in the U.S. & Canada)
314-447-8871 (subscribers outside of the U.S. & Canada)

Fax number: 314-447-8029

Elsevier Health Sciences Division
Subscription Customer Service
3251 Riverport Lane
Maryland Heights, MO 63043

*To ensure uninterrupted delivery of your subscription, please notify us at least 4 weeks in advance of move.

Printed and bound by CPI Group (UK) Ltd, Croydon, CR0 4YY

03/10/2024

01040453-0015